中医舌诊与临床研究
（汉英对照）

TCM Tongue Diagnosis and Clinical Research
(Chinese-English)

主　编　　丁成华

Chief Editors　Ding Chenghua

孙晓刚

Sun Xiaogang

中国中医药出版社

·北　京·

China Press of Traditional Chinese Medicine

· Beijing ·

图书在版编目（CIP）数据

中医舌诊与临床研究：汉英对照 / 丁成华，孙晓刚
主编 . —北京：中国中医药出版社，2019.12
ISBN 978-7-5132-5961-3

Ⅰ . ①中… Ⅱ . ①丁… ②孙… Ⅲ . ①舌诊—研究—
汉、英 Ⅳ . ① R241.25

中国版本图书馆 CIP 数据核字（2019）第 289226 号

中国中医药出版社出版

北京经济技术开发区科创十三街 31 号院二区 8 号楼
邮政编码　100176
传真　010-64405750
三河市同力彩印有限公司印刷
各地新华书店经销

开本 787×1092　1/16　印张 17　字数 466 千字
2019 年 12 月第 1 版　2019 年 12 月第 1 次印刷
书号　ISBN 978-7-5132-5961-3

定价　118.00 元
网址　www.cptcm.com

社 长 热 线　010-64405720
购 书 热 线　010-89535836
维 权 打 假　010-64405753

微信服务号　**zgzyycbs**
微商城网址　**https://kdt.im/LIdUGr**
官 方 微 博　**http://e.weibo.com/cptcm**
天猫旗舰店网址　**https://zgzyycbs.tmall.com**

如有印装质量问题请与本社出版部联系（010-64405510）
版权专有　侵权必究

前　言

Preface

舌诊是中医独具特色的诊断方法之一。舌象是观察人体生理病理的一个窗口，表征着人体健康与疾病状态。古语云："望而知之谓之神。"舌诊是中医望诊的重要内容之一，是临床诊治疾病的主要依据。

Tongue diagnosis is one of the unique diagnostic methods of Traditional Chinese Medicine (TCM). Tongue manifestation is a window to observe the human body physiologically and pathologically, which characterizes the body's healthy or sick state. As the old saying goes, "People who know the cause of the disease through inspection can be called immortals." Tongue diagnosis is one of the important contents of TCM inspection and the main basis of clinical diagnosis and treatment.

中医学认为人体是由脏腑、经络、形体、官窍构成的一个有机整体，它们之间在生理上相互关联，在病理上相互影响。舌通过经络、经筋与各脏腑相连属，脏腑气血津液之盛衰、脏腑气化功能之强弱，均反映于舌。临床实践证明，在疾病发展过程中，舌的变化迅速而明显，能较为客观地反映病位的浅深、病邪的性质、邪正的盛衰及病势的进退，是临床上辨证论治的重要依据。临证时，四诊合参，详辨舌象，是取得疗效的根本保证。

Traditional Chinese Medicine holds that the human body is an organic whole composed of *zang-fu* organs, meridians, physique, sensory organs and orifices, which are physiologically interrelated and affect each other pathologically. The tongue is connected with *zang-fu* organs through meridians, collaterals and sinews. Therefore, it can reflect the exuberance and debilitation of qi, blood, body fluid and qi transformation of different *zang-fu* organs.

1

Clinical practice shows that, in the process of disease development, tongue manifestation with rapid and obvious changes can objectively reflect the depth of the disease location, the nature of the pathogens, the wax and wane between the pathogens and healthy qi, and the condition of disease tendency, all of which are important basis for syndrome differentiation and treatment. Clinically, detailed inspection of tongue manifestation and comprehensive analysis of four diagnostic methods assure good curative effect.

本书内容涵盖舌诊概述、舌诊基础研究、舌诊临床应用三大部分，舌诊现代研究附后。全书334幅舌象照片、60例临床病案，均精选于作者团队长期在临床一线所采集的资料；内容翔实，图文并茂。

This book covers three parts: Overview of the Tongue Diagnosis, Basic Research of the Tongue Diagnosis and Clinical Application of the Tongue Diagnosis. Furthermore, the modern research on tongue diagnosis is attached. In this book, 334 tongue manifestations and 60 clinical cases were first-hand data collected by the author's team in clinic in a long duration, with vivid pictures and detailed contents.

第一章"舌诊概述"，对舌诊源流、舌诊原理、舌形态与生理功能、舌诊的临床意义进行了梳理。第二章"舌诊基础研究"，对舌质的神、色、形、态，舌苔的苔质、苔色，按舌象特征、临床意义、机理分析给予了详细介绍。第三章"舌诊临床应用"，首先对常见证候的主要症状与舌象特征逐证归纳整理；其次对临证中具有典型舌象特征，治疗前后舌象有明显变化的心、肝、脾、肺、肾五大系统病案各12例予以重点阐述，并力求舌象典型、图像清晰，文字简练、表述准确，病案具有代表性。各案例在临证中，既四诊合参，条分缕析，详细辨证，又有针对性地辨析舌象与相关病、证、症之间的内在关联性，从四诊确定证型、病名，从舌象佐证病、证，从而确立处方用药的原则与方法；复诊时根据患者四诊信息及舌象变化，调整治疗方案及处方用药与剂量，体现一理一法皆有据可凭，一方一药均有的放矢；案后证候分析，法扣医理，且突出中医舌诊的独特作用。第四章总结了近10年的舌诊有关研究成果。

The first Chapter of "Overview of the Tongue Diagnosis" illustrates systematically the origin of tongue diagnosis, the principle of tongue diagnosis, the morphology and physiological functions of the tongue, and the clinical significance of tongue diagnosis.

The second Chapter of "Basic Research of the Tongue Diagnosis" gives a detailed introduction to the spirit, color, form and movement of the tongue as well as the texture and color of tongue fur. Clinical significance and mechanism of tongue manifestation had been given according to the characteristics.

In the third Chapter of "Clinical Application of the Tongue Diagnosis", firstly, the main symptoms and tongue manifestation characteristics of common syndromes are summarized one by one. Secondly, it focuses on the 12 representative cases of the five systems of heart, liver, spleen, lung and kidney, which have typical features of the tongue manifestation and obvious manifestation changes before and after treatment. All cases are illustrated with clear pictures, concise text and accurate descriptions.

Each case in clinic not only shows comprehensive analysis of four diagnostic methods and systematic syndrome differentiation but also distinguishes the intrinsic relationship between tongue manifestation with related diseases, patterns and symptoms. On this basis, disease and its syndromes are confirmed by four diagnostic methods and collaboratively proved by tongue manifestation, thus, the principles and methods of prescription and medication are decided. In following-up visits, the treatment, prescription and dosage will be adjusted according to the patient's four-examination information and tongue manifestation changes to embody the flexibility of principle-method-recipe-medicinal. The comment on the medical record is closely combined with the method and the theory, highlighting the unique role of tongue diagnosis.

The last part summarizes the research results of tongue diagnosis in recent 10 years.

笔者从事中医教学、科研、临床工作 30 余年，深感中医舌诊在观察人体生命活动和疾病变化的实践中独具特色，折射出中国传统文化整体观、辩证观、恒动观、中和观及象思维等深邃的东方哲学智慧。全书设中英文对照，有利于中医文化的对外交流。希冀中外好医者有所得，从而能够登堂入室，将中医瑰宝发扬光大。然精益求精，尤有不及，疏漏之处，就正方家。

I have been engaging in TCM teaching, scientific research and clinical work for more than 30 years, and deeply feels that, in observing human life activities and disease changes, tongue diagnosis is unique that reflects the profound eastern philosophical wisdom in Chinese traditional culture such as the concepts of holism, dialecticism, constant movement, golden mean and image thinking. The Chinese-English version facilitates the foreign exchange of TCM culture. I hope that the practitioners at home and abroad will be benefited from this book and become more proficient, so as to carry forward the treasures of Traditional Chinese Medicine. Hard as we tried, there are surely some flaws that need the suggestion and criticism from experts.

感谢参与本书编写的全体成员；感谢江西中医药大学附属医院主任医师胡珂、梁启军、伍建光、宋卫国，江西省人民医院主任医师陈耀辉，南昌大学第三附属医院丁明、方华珍老师及南昌大学第四附属医院万悦老师参与或协助临床资料的采集工作；感谢就读于江西中医药大学已毕业和在读的博、硕研究生参与本书临床资料的收集整理工作：王河宝、齐城成、高秀娟、尚姝、盘莉、方华珍、曹晓瑞、冯磊、马丽珍、兰佳、陈雪姣、王玉臣、宁伦、张珂、林霖、高巍巍、陈玲、邓露露、李伟、张伟、钟爱萍、王瑞、徐丽、周灵情、何愉、董艳玉、李石林、石国栋、李琪、袁丽霞。

Thanks to all the members who participated in the preparation of this book, including Hu Ke, Liang Qijun, Wu Jianguang, Song Weiguo, chief physicians of the Affiliated Hospital of Jiangxi University of TCM; Chen Yaohui, chief physician of Jiangxi Provincial People's Hospital; Ding Ming and Fang Huazhen, from the Third Affiliated Hospital of Nanchang University; Wan Yue, from the Fourth Affiliated Hospital of Nanchang University; Wang Hebao, Qi Chengcheng, Gao Xiujuan, Shang Shu, Pan li, Fang Huazhen, Cao Xiaorui, Feng Lei, Ma Lizhen, Lan Jia, Chen Xuejiao, Wang Yuchen, Ning Lun, Zhang Ke, Lin lin, Gao Weiwei, Chen Ling, Deng Lulu, Li Wei, Zhang Wei, Zhong Aiping, Wang Rui, Xu Li, Zhou Lingqing, He Yu, Dong Yanyu, Li Shilin, Shi Guodong, Li Qi, Yuan Lixia, previous or present postgraduates from Jiangxi University of TCM.

感谢中国中医药出版社本书责编单宝枝主任的精心指导。

Thanks for the meticulous guidance of Shan Baozhi, executive editor of China Press of Traditional Chinese Medicine.

本书受国家自然科学基金项目（81260527，81760842），国家精品课程（教高函〔2010〕14号），国家精品资源共享课程（教高函〔2016〕54号），国家中医药管理局重点学科（国中医药人教发〔2012〕32号），江西省高校人文社会科学研究项目（JY162051），江西省研究生优质课程（赣教办函〔2016〕95号）资助，在此表示感谢。

This book is funded by the National Natural Science Foundation of China (No.81260527, No.81760842), the National Top-Quality Course (Higher Education

Division of Ministry of Education〔2010〕No.14), the National Top-Quality Resources-Sharing Course (Higher Education Division of Ministry of Education〔2016〕No.54), the Key Discipline of State Administration of TCM (Personnel Education Division of State Administration of TCM〔2012〕No.32), the Humanities and Social Sciences Project for Higher-Learning Institutions in Jiangxi Province (No.JY162051), the Excellent Course for Postgraduates in Jiangxi Province (Jiangxi Provincial Department of Education〔2016〕No.95). Thanks for all the support.

丁成华

Ding Chenghua

2019 年 1 月于江西中医药大学

Jiangxi University of Traditional Chinese Medicine

January, 2019

目　录

Contents

第一章　舌诊概述
Chapter 1　Overview of the Tongue Diagnosis

第一节　舌诊的发展源流 ·················· 3
Section 1　Origin and Development of the Tongue Diagnosis ·············· 3

第二节　舌的形态结构与生理功能 ·················· 7
Section 2　Shape and Structures and Physiological Function of Tongue ·············· 7

一、形态结构 ·················· 7

1. Shape and structure

二、生理功能 ·················· 9

2. Physiological function

第三节　舌诊原理 ·················· 10
Section 3　Mechanism of Tongue Diagnosis

一、舌与脏腑经络的关系 ·················· 10

1. Relationship between tongue, viscera and meridians

二、舌与气血津液的关系 ·················· 10

2. Relationship between tongue and qi, blood, body fluid

三、舌面与脏腑的对应关系 ·················· 11

3. Correspondence of the tongue to the viscera

第四节　舌诊的临床意义 ·················· 12
Section 4　Clinical Significance of the Tongue Diagnosis

一、判断邪正盛衰 ·················· 12

1. To judge the exuberance or debilitation of the vital-qi and the pathogenic-qi

二、区别病邪性质 ·· 14

2. To distinguish the nature of disease pathogen

三、判别病位浅深 ·· 15

3. To detect the shallow or deep location of disease

四、推断病势进退 ·· 17

4. To infer the tendency of disease

五、估计病情预后 ·· 21

5. To estimate the prognosis of disease

第二章　舌诊基础研究

Chapter 2　Basic Research of the Tongue Diagnosis

第一节　诊舌质 ·· 25

Section 1　Inspection of Tongue Texture

一、舌神 ·· 25

1.Tongue vitality (Spirit)

（一）有神（荣舌）·· 25

1.1　Full vitality（Luxuriant tongue）

（二）无神（枯舌）·· 26

1.2　Lacking of vitality（Withered tongue）

二、舌色 ·· 26

2. Tongue color

（一）淡红舌 ·· 26

2.1　Pink tongue

（二）淡白舌 ·· 28

2.2　Pale tongue

（三）红舌 ·· 29

2.3　Red tongue

（四）绛舌 ·· 31

2.4　Crimson Tongue

（五）青紫舌 ……………………………… 32

2.5　Bluish purple tongue

三、舌形 …………………………………… 34

3.Tongue shape

（一）老、嫩舌 …………………………… 34

3.1　Tough and tender tongue

（二）胖、瘦舌 …………………………… 35

3.2　Enlarged and thin tongue

（三）齿痕舌 ……………………………… 37

3.3　Teeth-marked tongue

（四）点、刺舌 …………………………… 38

3.4　Pointed and pricked tongue

（五）裂纹舌 ……………………………… 40

3.5　Fissured tongue

四、舌态 …………………………………… 41

4. Tongue motility

（一）痿软舌 ……………………………… 41

4.1　Flaccid tongue

（二）强硬舌 ……………………………… 42

4.2　Stiff tongue

（三）歪斜舌 ……………………………… 43

4.3　Deviated tongue

（四）吐弄舌 ……………………………… 43

4.4　Protruding and waggling tongue

（五）短缩舌 ……………………………… 44

4.5　Shortened tongue

（六）颤动舌 ……………………………… 45

4.6　Trembling tongue

五、舌下络脉 ……………………………… 46

5. Sublingual veins

（一）正常舌脉 …………………………… 46

5.1　Normal tongue vein

（二）异常舌脉 ··· 46

5.2　Abnormal tongue vein

第二节　诊舌苔 ··· 48

Section 2　Inspection of the Tongue Fur

一、苔质 ··· 48

1. Tongue fur texture

（一）厚、薄苔 ··· 48

1.1　Thick and thin fur

（二）润、燥苔 ··· 49

1.2　Moist and dry tongue fur

（三）腻、腐苔 ··· 51

1.3　Slimy and curdy fur

（四）剥落苔 ··· 52

1.4　Peeled fur

（五）偏、全苔 ··· 55

1.5　Tongue fur covered on full or part of tongue body

（六）真、假苔 ··· 56

1.6　True and false tongue fur

二、苔色 ··· 57

2. Inspection of the color of the tongue fur

（一）白苔 ··· 57

2.1　White fur

（二）黄苔 ··· 59

2.2　Yellow fur

（三）灰黑苔 ··· 63

2.3　Gray-black fur

第三章　舌诊临床应用

Chapter 3　Clinical Application of the Tongue Diagnosis

第一节　常见证候的舌象特征 ·· 67

Section 1　Tongue Manifestation Characteristics of Common Syndrome

一、气虚证 ·· 67

1. Qi deficiency syndrome

二、血虚证 ·· 68

2. Blood deficiency syndrome

三、阴虚证 ·· 69

3. Yin deficiency syndrome

四、阳虚证 ·· 70

4. Yang deficiency syndrome

五、津液亏虚证 ·· 71

5. Fluid and humor deficiency syndrome

六、气滞证 ·· 72

6. Qi stagnation syndrome

七、血瘀证 ·· 73

7. Blood stasis syndrome

八、实热证 ·· 74

8. Excess heat syndrome

九、实寒证 ·· 76

9. Excess cold syndrome

十、痰湿证 ·· 77

10. Phlegm-dampness syndrome

十一、食积证 ·· 79

11. Food accumulation syndrome

第二节　临床病证举隅 ·· 80

Section 2　Examples of Clinical Medical Records

一、心系病证 ·· 80

1. Heart System Syndrome

（一）心悸－心阳不足证 ···················· 80

1.1　Palpitation: syndrome of heart yang deficiency

（二）心悸－心阳虚衰证 ···················· 82

1.2　Palpitation: syndrome of heart yang debilitation

（三）心悸－心阴亏虚证 ···················· 84

1.3　Palpitation: syndrome of heart yin deficiency

（四）心悸－气虚血瘀证 ···················· 87

1.4　Palpitation: syndrome of qi deficiency and blood stasis

（五）心悸－心胆气虚证 ···················· 89

1.5　Palpitation: syndrome of qi deficiency of heart and gallbladder

（六）心悸－湿热浸淫证 ···················· 91

1.6　Palpitation: syndrome of dampness-heat intrusion and spreading

（七）不寐－心脾两虚证 ···················· 93

1.7　Insomnia: syndrome of dual deficiency of heart and spleen

（八）不寐－心肾不交证 ···················· 95

1.8　Insomnia: syndrome of non-interaction between heart and kidney

（九）胸痹－气滞血瘀证 ···················· 97

1.9　Chest impediment: syndrome of qi stagnation and blood stasis

（十）胸痹－心脉瘀阻证 ···················· 100

1.10　Chest impediment: syndrome of heart stasis obstruction

（十一）胸痹－痰瘀互结证 ···················· 102

1.11　Chest impediment: syndrome of phlegm and stasis binding

（十二）胸痹－痰瘀互结证 ···················· 104

1.12　Chest impediment: syndrome of phlegm and stasis binding

二、肝胆系病证 ···················· 107

2. Liver and gallbladder system syndrome

（一）胁痛－肝胆湿热证　···················· 107

2.1　Hypochondriac pain: syndrome of dampness-heat in the liver and gallbladder

（二）胁痛－肝胆湿热证 ···················· 109

2.2　Hypochondriac pain: syndrome of dampness-heat in the liver and gallbladder

（三）胁胀－肝肾阴虚证 ···················· 111

2.3　Hypochondriac pain: syndrome of yin deficiency of liver and kidney

（四）胁胀－肝胆湿热证 ·················· 114

2.4　Hypochondriac distention: syndrome of dampness-heat in the liver and gallbladder

（五）奔豚气－肝郁气滞证 ·················· 116

2.5　Running piglet qi: syndrome of liver depression and qi stagnation

（六）积聚－湿热蕴结证 ·················· 118

2.6　Abdominal mass: syndrome of dampness-heat accumulation

（七）臌胀－水湿困脾证 ·················· 120

2.7　Tympanites: syndrome of water-dampness encumbering spleen

（八）郁证－肝郁气滞证 ·················· 123

2.8　Depression: syndrome of liver depression and qi stagnation

（九）黄疸－热重于湿证 ·················· 125

2.9　Jaundice: syndrome of predominance of heat over dampness

（十）头痛－寒滞肝经证 ·················· 127

2.10　Headache: syndrome of cold stagnating in the liver meridian

（十一）转筋－肝络失养证 ·················· 129

2.11　Twitch: symptom of insufficient nourishment of liver collateral

（十二）震颤－肝肾阴虚证 ·················· 131

2.12　Tremor: syndrome of yin deficiency of liver and kidney

三、脾胃系病证 ·················· 134

3. Spleen and stomach disease syndrome

（一）胃痛－心脾两虚证 ·················· 134

3.1　Stomachache: syndrome of deficiency of both heart and spleen

（二）胃痛－肝气犯胃证 ·················· 136

3.2　Stomachache: syndrome of liver qi invading stomach

（三）胃痛－湿热内蕴证 ·················· 139

3.3　Stomachache: syndrome of internal accumulation of dampness-heat

（四）胃痞－肝郁脾虚证 ·················· 141

3.4　Stomach stuffiness: syndrome of liver depression and spleen deficiency

（五）胃痞－脾虚湿困证 ·················· 143

3.5　Stomach stuffiness: syndrome of spleen deficiency and dampness encumbering

（六）胃痞 – 脾气亏虚证 ·· 146

3.6 Stomach stuffiness: syndrome of depleting spleen qi

（七）腹胀 – 肝郁化火证 ·· 148

3.7 Abdominal distension: syndrome of liver depression transforming into fire

（八）嘈杂 – 脾胃虚弱证 ·· 150

3.8 Epigastric upset: syndrome of deficiency of spleen and stomach

（九）腹泻 – 气虚外感证 ·· 152

3.9 Diarrhea: syndrome of qi deficiency and external contraction

（十）便秘 – 阳虚证 ·· 154

3.10 Constipation: syndrome of yang deficiency

（十一）呃逆 – 气虚证 ·· 156

3.11 Hiccup: qi deficiency symptom

（十二）呕吐 – 肝气犯胃证 ·· 158

3.12 Vomiting: syndrome of liver qi invading stomach

四、肺系病证 ··· 160

4. Respiratory disease syndrome

（一）咳嗽 – 风寒袭肺证 ·· 160

4.1 Cough: syndrome of wind-cold fettering lung

（二）咳嗽 – 痰湿壅肺证 ·· 162

4.2 Cough: syndrome of phlegm-dampness obstructing lung

（三）咳嗽 – 痰热壅肺证 ·· 165

4.3 Cough: syndrome of phlegm-heat obstructing lung

（四）喘证 – 肺气虚证 ·· 167

4.4 Dyspnea: syndrome of qi deficiency of lung

（五）喘证 – 痰热蕴肺证 ·· 170

4.5 Dyspnea: syndrome of phlegm-heat accumulating lung

（六）哮喘 – 肺脾气虚证 ·· 172

4.6 Asthma: syndrome of qi deficiency of lung and spleen

（七）哮证 – 冷哮证 ·· 174

4.7 Wheezing: cold wheezing syndrome

（八）肺胀 – 痰湿蕴肺证 ·· 176

4.8　Lung distention: syndrome of phlegm-dampness accumulating lung

（九）乳蛾－肺经风热证 ·································· 178

4.9　Tonsillitis: syndrome of wind-heat in lung meridian

（十）肺痈－痰热蕴肺证 ·································· 180

4.10　Lung abscess: syndrome of phlegm-heat accumulating lung

（十一）失音－肺燥津伤证 ······························ 182

4.11　Aphonia: syndrome of lung dryness damaging fluid

（十二）咯血－肝火犯肺证 ······························ 184

4.12　Hemoptysis: syndrome of liver fire invading lung

五、肾系病证 ·· 186

5. Kidney system syndrome

（一）水肿－脾肾阳虚证 ·································· 186

5.1　Edema: syndrome of yang deficiency of spleen and kidney

（二）水肿－脾肾阳虚证 ·································· 188

5.2　Edema: syndrome of yang deficiency of spleen and kidney

（三）水肿－脾肾气虚证 ·································· 190

5.3　Edema: syndrome of qi deficiency of spleen and kidney

（四）水肿－脾肾气虚证 ·································· 193

5.4　Edema: syndrome of spleen-kidney qi deficiency

（五）水肿－肾气亏虚证 ·································· 195

5.5　Edema: syndrome of kidney qi deficiency

（六）淋证－肾阴不足，湿热下注证 ···················· 197

5.6　Stranguria: syndrome of kidney yin deficiency and dampness-heat pouring downward

（七）淋证－湿热内阻证 ·································· 199

5.7　Stranguria: syndrome of internal obstruction of dampness-heat

（八）石淋－湿热内蕴证 ·································· 202

5.8　Stone stranguria: syndrome of dampness-heat accumulation

（九）血淋－湿热下注证 ·································· 204

5.9　Blood strangury: syndrome of dampness-heat flowing downward

（十）尿浊－脾肾气虚证 ·································· 206

5.10　Turbid urine: syndrome of qi deficiency of spleen and kidney

（十一）消渴－肾阴亏虚证 ···················· 208

5.11　Consumptive thirst: syndrome of kidney yin deficiency

（十二）消渴－肾阴阳两虚证 ···················· 210

5.12　Consumptive thirst: syndrome of deficiency of both yin and yang of kidney

第四章　舌诊研究进展

Chapter 4　Research Progress of the Tongue Diagnosis

第一节　舌诊临床应用研究 ···················· 215

Section 1　Research on the Clinical Application of Tongue Diagnosis

一、舌诊在肝系疾病中的应用 ···················· 215

1. Application of tongue diagnosis in liver diseases

二、舌诊在心系疾病的应用 ···················· 217

2. Application of tongue diagnosis in heart diseases

三、舌诊在脾胃系疾病的应用 ···················· 220

3. Application of tongue diagnosis in spleen-stomach diseases

四、舌诊在肺系疾病的应用 ···················· 221

4. Application of tongue diagnosis in lung diseases

五、舌诊在肾系疾病的应用 ···················· 223

5. Application of tongue diagnosis in kidney diseases

第二节　舌诊的实验研究 ···················· 225

Section 2　Experimental Research of Tongue Diagnosis

一、科学仪器的检测研究 ···················· 225

1. Detection research of scientific instruments

二、分子生物学技术的舌诊研究 ···················· 226

2. Tongue diagnosis research of molecular biology technique

三、光谱分析法 ···················· 227

3. Spectral analysis method

四、高光谱图分析法 ···················· 229

4. Hyperspectral graph analysis method

第三节 舌诊的客观化研究 ·············· 230
Section 3　Objective Study of Tongue Diagnosis

一、计算机技术研究舌诊图像 ·············· 230

1. Tongue diagnosis image based on computer technology

二、舌诊仪研究 ·············· 232

2. Study on tongue diagnosis instrument

三、舌质的客观化研究 ·············· 234

3. Study on objectification of tongue texture

四、舌苔的客观化研究 ·············· 236

4. Study on objectification of tongue fur

参考文献 ·············· 239
References

第一章 舌诊概述

Chapter 1　Overview of the Tongue Diagnosis

舌诊是中医四诊的重要内容之一，在中医辨证论治中发挥着极其重要的作用。历代医家在长期的医疗实践中，认识到舌象的变化与疾病的发生发展存在着密切联系，经过反复观察、论证，形成了独具特色的中医舌诊理论与方法。

Tongue diagnosis, one of the important contents of four diagnostic methods in Traditional Chinese Medicine (TCM), plays an extremely important role in TCM syndrome differentiation and treatment. During the long-term medical practice, generations of physicians realized that the tongue manifestation changes were closely related to the occurrence and development of the diseases. After repeated observation and confirmation, the unique theory and method of TCM tongue diagnosis had been formed.

第一节　舌诊的发展源流

Section 1　Origin and Development of the Tongue Diagnosis

中医舌诊历史悠久，早在殷墟甲骨文中就有"贞疾舌"的记载。成书于两千多年前的《黄帝内经》已经有舌诊的描述，如《灵枢·经脉》曰："手少阴之别……循经入于心中，系舌本。"《素问·刺热》记载："肺热病者……舌上黄。"充分证明，当时对舌象的生理病理已有一定的认识，对后世舌诊研究有重要影响。

Tongue diagnosis has a very long history with the record of "diagnosing morbid tongue" on *Yinxu* oracle bone inscriptions of the Shang dynasty. And there are already descriptions of the tongue diagnosis in the book *The Yellow Emperor's Inner Classic* written more than 2000 years ago. For example, *The Spiritual Pivot-Meridians* recorded that "The divergence of heart meridian of hand-shaoyin... goes through the heart and links with the tongue"; *The Plain Question- Acupuncture on Heat Syndrome* stated: "Syndrome of lung heat ... would show the yellow tongue." This fully proved that the physiology and pathology of the tongue had been understood partly then, which has an important effect on tongue diagnosis in later generations.

东汉张仲景继承《黄帝内经》的舌诊理论，并在临证实践中予以发展，使舌诊在理论和内容上都有了较大的发展。在《伤寒杂病论》中有不少关于舌诊内容的详细记载，并运用舌象进行辨证，审察病因，阐述病机，确定治则，判断预后。汉代另一大医家华佗在《中藏经》中也有关于舌与脏腑之间关系的记载，如"阳厥论第四"中有"咽干口焦，舌生疮"，"论肝脏虚实寒热生死逆顺脉证之法第二十二"有"肝中寒则两臂痛不能举，舌本燥"。充分表明，舌诊在汉代已经作为疾病诊断的重要内容之一。

In the Eastern Han dynasty, based on the inheritance of the tongue diagnosis theory in *The Yellow Emperor's Inner Classic,* Zhang Zhongjing made new important contribution to its development in the clinical practices.

There are many detailed records about tongue diagnosis in the book *Treatise on Febrile and Miscellaneous Diseases*, and tongue manifestations are used for syndrome differentiation, cause examination, pathogenesis elaboration, treatment determination and prognosis judgment.

Hua Tuo, another famous doctor in the Han dynasty, also described the relationship between tongue and *zang-fu* organs in *Central Treasury Classic*. For example, in the Section "On Yang Syncope, the Fourth", it recorded that "Dry pharyngeal and scorched mouth, with sores on the tongue"; and in the Section "On Pulse and Syndrome of Deficiency and Excess, Cold and Heat, Life and Death, and Favorable and Unfavorable, the Twenty-second", it stated that "Cold invasion of the liver induces dry tongue and pain in both arms with failure to lift up"; which fully showed that tongue diagnosis has already been an important part of disease diagnosis in the Han dynasty.

晋代皇甫谧在《针灸甲乙经》中记述了针灸治疗舌缓、重舌、舌不能言、舌下肿、舌纵等病症。晋代王叔和在舌诊立论方面有新的见解，如《脉经·热病十逆死证篇》中曰："热病七八日……舌焦干黑者死。""热病身面尽黄而肿，心热口干，舌卷焦黄黑……伏毒伤肺中脾者死。"晋代葛洪在《肘后救卒方》记载了十余条有关舌诊的内容。如在"治伤寒时气瘟病篇"中有"若病人齿无色，舌上白，或喜睡眠，愦愦不知痛痒处。"

In the Jin dynasty, Huangfu Mi described the acupuncture treatment of slacken tongue, double tongue, tongue dysfunction impeding speech, sublingual swelling, protracted tongue and other diseases in *The Systematic Classic of Acupuncture and Moxibustion*.

New ideas were put forward by Wang Shuhe in theory. For example, in the book *The Pulse Classic-Ten Unfavorable and Fatal Syndrome of Febrile Disease*, it stated that "febrile disease for seven or eight days... the patient will die with the scorched, dry and black tongue." "yellow skin and complexion with swelling, heat heart and dry mouth, curled and scorched tongue with yellow and black colors... the patient will die from latent toxin attacking lung and spleen."

The book *Emergency Formulas to Keep Up One's Sleeve* by Ge Hong in the Jin dynasty recorded more than ten articles of tongue diagnosis. For example, in the Section "Treatment to Cold Damage, Seasonal Qi and Pestilent Disease", it recorded that "for the patient with lusterless teeth, pale tongue, or drowsiness and imperception to pain and itch."

隋代巢元方在《诸病源候论》中重视察舌以寻诸病之源，对舌肿、舌胀、舌卷、舌烂、舌不收、重舌等舌态进行了详细描述；对舌色也有论述，如舌上白、舌上黄、舌上白黄、舌赤等。同时，巢氏在"噤黄候"中曰："身面发黄，舌下大脉起青黑色，舌噤强不能语，名为噤黄也。"这是第一次对舌下络脉进行诊断。

In the Sui dynasty, Chao Yuanfang in the book *Treatise on the Origins and Manifestations of Various Diseases* attached importance to observe the tongues to find the origins of the diseases. The form, movement and color of the tongue were also described in details in the book, such as swollen tongue, distending tongue, curled tongue, rotten tongue, protrusive tongue, double tongue, white tongue fur, yellow tongue fur, white-yellow tongue fur, and red tongue, etc. Chao also described "the symptom of clenched jaundice" with the statement that "The symptom of yellow skin and complexion, cyanotic black sublingual vessels, clenched and stiff tongue impeding speech is called clenched jaundice (jaundice with dysphagia)" . This is the first record on the diagnosis of the sublingual vessels.

唐代的舌诊研究与临床应用也有明显进步，唐代大医家孙思邈在《备急千金要方》中专门写下"舌论"一章，总结前代医家对舌诊的论述，同时也为后世的舌诊给予启迪与开拓。如他辨脏腑以察舌质为主，较巢元方的重视舌体变化又进了一步。唐代王焘在《外台秘要》中提出舌与人所食五味的关系，如"若多食咸，则舌脉凝而变色。多食苦，则皮槁而毛拔。多食辛，则舌筋急而枯干"。

Great progress of tongue diagnosis and its clinical application had also been made in the Tang dynasty. Sun Simiao purposefully wrote the Chapter *Treatise on the Tongue* in the book *Important Formulas Worth a Thousand Gold Pieces* to summarize the discussions on tongue diagnosis in previous generations and also provide enlightenment and exploration for tongue diagnosis in later generations. For example, Sun mainly focused on tongue texture to distinguish the viscera disease, which was a further step forward than Chao Yuanfang's emphasis on the changes of tongue body. Moreover, Wang Tao put forward the relationship between the tongue and five flavors in the book *Arcane Essentials from the Imperial Library*. For example, it stated that "Excessive taking of salty food stagnates the tongue blood vessels and change the complexion. Excessive taking of bitter food makes the skin dry and body hair lose. Excessive taking of pungent food causes dryness and cramp of tongue tendons."

宋、金、元时期，医学肇兴，学术争鸣，医学界理论不断创新，各家竞相立说，舌诊学也得到充分发展。金元四大家的著作中都体现了他们对察舌辨证的实践和不同见解，为舌诊的发展起到了承前启后的作用。公元 1341 年，我国第一部舌诊专著——《敖氏伤寒金镜录》问世。该书原本以 12 舌图验证、论说伤寒表里，后经杜清碧增补 24 图，合为 36 图，并在图下列出治则与方药，使其趋于完善。

During the Song, Jin and Yuan dynasties, medicine developed and flourished with continuous innovation and establishment of medical theories, and tongue diagnosis was also fully developed. Four representatives of Jin and Yuan dynasties had different insight and practice in tongue diagnosis and syndrome differentiation in their respective works, which was a bridge between the past and the future. In 1341 A.D., China's first tongue diagnostic monograph *Ao's Golden Mirror Records for Cold Damage* came out. The book originally had 12 tongue pictures to verify and explain the internal and external syndromes of cold damage. Later, Du Qingbi added 24 tongue pictures (36 pictures in total) and completed them better with therapeutic principles and prescriptions after the pictures.

明清时期，随着温病学的兴起与发展，辨舌验齿更加得到重视。如戴天章发展以舌分辨瘟疫与伤寒；叶天士在《瘟疫论》中注重辨舌验齿，将舌诊运用到卫气营血的辨证当中；吴鞠通在《温病条辨》中将舌诊与三焦辨证有机结合起来，对舌苔的色泽、舌津盈亏、舌色深浅、舌体强弱等方面进行论述，从而确立了温病察舌辨证施治的原则。

With the development of Warm Diseases Theory during the Ming and Qing dynasties, the observation and examination of tongue and tooth got more and more attention. For example, Dai Tianzhang diagnosed the pestilence and cold attack based on tongue diagnosis; in the *Treatise on Warm-Heat Pestilence*, Ye Tianshi valued the observation and examination of tongue and tooth, and applied tongue diagnosis to syndrome differentiation of defensive-qi-nutrient-blood; Wu Jutong, in the book *Systematic Differentiation of Warm Diseases*, combined tongue diagnosis and syndrome differentiation of triple energizer, and expounded such aspects as the color and lustre of the tongue, sufficiency and insufficiency of the tongue fluid, darkness and lightness of the color, strength and weakness of the tongue body, thus, established the therapeutic principle for warm and febrile diseases, namely, the principle of syndrome differentiation and treatment through tongue diagnosis.

民国时期，曹炳章著有《辨舌指南》，附彩图 122 幅、墨图 6 幅，以现代医学的解剖、组织、生理学来阐明中医舌诊的原理，汇集整理了历代医家有关舌诊的重要理论，为近代舌诊研究提供知识宝库。新中国成立以来，舌诊研究方兴未艾，无论在微观还是宏观均取得了极大进步。相信随着科技的进步，以及多学科的交汇发展，中医舌诊的研究将会迈向更广阔的发展空间。

In the period of the Republic of China, Cao Bingzhang published the book *Guide to Tongue Diagnosis*, with 122 color drawings and 6 black-white drawings of tongues. Cao illustrated tongue diagnosis theory by modern anatomy, histology and physiology, compiled tongue diagnosis theories of generations of physicians and provided a treasury of knowledge for tongue diagnosis research in modern times. Since the founding of new China, the study of tongue diagnosis has been booming and great progress has been made in both micro and macro aspects. It is believed that the research of TCM tongue diagnosis will meet a promising future with scientific and technological advancement as well as multi-disciplinary convergence.

第二节　舌的形态结构与生理功能

Section 2　Shape and Structures and Physiological Function of Tongue

一、形态结构
1. Shape and structure

舌是由黏膜和舌肌组成的肌性器官，它附着于口腔底部、下颌骨、舌骨，呈扁平长形状。舌的上面称舌背，下面称舌底（图 1.2.1.1，图 1.2.1.2）。舌背又分为舌体与舌根两部分，以人字沟为分界。舌体的前端称为舌尖，舌体的后部人字形界沟之前称为舌根，舌体的中部称为舌中，舌体的两侧称为舌边，舌面的正中有一条不甚明显的纵行皱褶，称为舌正中沟（图 1.2.1.3）。

The Tongue, a muscular organ made up of mucous membranes and tongue muscles, is attached by muscles to the lower jawbone and hyoid bone. It is flat and long. The feature of tongue includes tongue back and tongue bottom. Tongue back is divided into two part—tongue body and tongue root (Fig.1.2.1.1, Fig.1.2.1.2), which are bordered by a gulf in middle surface of tongue, shaped-like "人". Anterior tongue is called tongue tip. While the posterior is known as tongue root, the middle of tongue is tongue-middle and the margins of tongue is described tongue-margin. There is a vague striation in the middle of the surface of tongue, which is defined as tongue-middle-gulf (Fig.1.2.1.3).

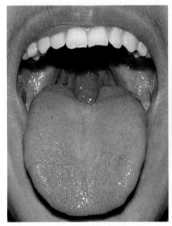 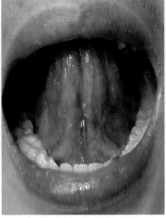 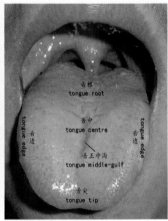

图 1.2.1.1
Fig. 1.2.1.1

图 1.2.1.2
Fig. 1.2.1.2

图 1.2.1.3
Fig. 1.2.1.3

舌上卷时，可看到舌底。舌底正中线上有一条连于口腔底的皱襞，叫舌系带。舌系带左右两侧，有两根较粗大的舌下静脉，称为舌下络脉（图 1.2.1.4）。

When tongue winds upward, its bottom was seen. A ruga in the middle boundary of it, that attached the bottom of buccal cavity, is called frenulum of tongue. There are two long hypoglossal vessels, both on sides of the frenulum of tongue (Fig.1.2.1.4).

舌面上覆盖着一层半透明的黏膜，舌背黏膜粗糙，形成许多突起，构成舌乳头。根据形状不同，舌乳头分为丝状乳头、蕈状乳头、轮廓乳头和叶状乳头四种。其中丝状乳头与蕈状乳头对舌象的形成有着密切的联系，轮廓乳头、叶状乳头与味觉有关（图 1.2.1.5）。

Tongue is covered with a layer of semitransparent mucous membrane, which is very rough on its back. A series of cone-shaped small projections called tongue papillae is located on the tongue back too. There are four kinds papillae: filiform papillae, fungiform papillae, circumvallate papillae and foliate papillae. The first two play important role in forming tongue pictures, while the latter two have connection with sense of taste (Fig.1.2.1.5).

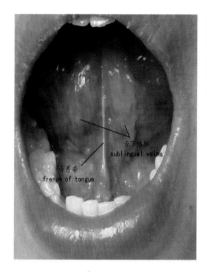

图 1.2.1.4
Fig. 1.2.1.4

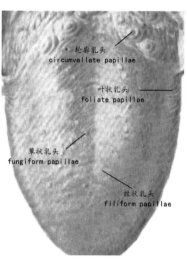

图 1.2.1.5
Fig. 1.2.1.5

二、生理功能
2. Physiological function

舌具有搅拌食物，感受味觉和调节语音的功能。舌作为一个肌性器官，能自主灵活地伸缩卷转，使食物在口腔内得到充分的搅拌。舌的轮廓乳头和叶状乳头内含味觉神经末梢，能充分感受味觉。舌的灵活自主运动，能配合胸腔、声带的发音，使语音清晰流畅。

Tongue has function of stirring food, feeling taste and regulating voice. As a muscular organ, the tongue can move smartly, as a result, food can be masticated throughout in the buccal cavity. In addition, there are lots of nerves endings in the out circumvallate papillae and foliate papillae, which helps the tongue to feel the taste completely. The smart movement of the tongue make speech clearly and fluently with support of the thorax and vocal cords.

第三节　舌诊原理

Section 3　Mechanism of Tongue Diagnosis

一、舌与脏腑经络的关系

1. Relationship between tongue, viscera and meridians

舌主要是通过经络与脏腑相关联。《灵枢·经脉》曰："手少阴之别……循经入于心中，系舌本。""肝者筋之合也，筋者，聚于阴器，而络于舌本也。""脾足太阴之脉……连舌本，散舌下。""肾足少阴之脉……其直者，从肾上贯肝膈，入肺中，循咽喉，夹舌本。"内脏都直接或间接与舌相联系。

The tongue connects the viscera with the help of the meridians. The book *The Spiritual Pivot-Meridians* recorded that "The divergence of heart meridian of hand-shaoyin... goes through the heart and links with the tongue." "The liver corresponds to the tendons that assemble on urethra and genitals, and links with the tongue." "Spleen meridian of foot-taiyin links the tongue." "Kidney meridian of foot-shaoyin goes upward and rounds the diaphragm, passes through the long, cross the throat and links the tongue." Obviously, the internal organs are directly or indirectly associated with the tongue.

二、舌与气血津液的关系

2. Relationship between tongue and qi, blood, body fluid

心主血为五脏六腑之大主，脾藏营而为诸脏后天之本。舌为心之苗窍、脾之外候，故诸脏营血之盈亏必显于舌。舌上之苔，为胃气熏蒸水谷浊气上潮所生，诸腑气化之动静亦易显于苔。另外，舌下有金津玉液，为胃津肾液上潮之孔道，如《灵枢·胀论》所曰："廉泉玉英者，津液之道也。"故津液之多少，亦显现于舌。舌体的形质与舌色与气血盈亏和运行状态有关，舌苔和舌体的润燥与津液的多少有关。

The heart dominates the blood and it's the supreme monarch of all organs. The spleen stores the nutritive blood and it's the foundation of acquired constitution. The tongue is the sprout of the heart and out-shows of the spleen. So the wax and wane of the nutrient and blood of *zang*-organs can be manifested by tongue. Tongue fur, produced by stomach qi fumigating the turbid qi of water and food and moistening of stomach fluid, exhibits the state of qi transformation of *fu*-organs. Besides, under the tongue are the pores- *Jinjin* and *Yuye* -through which the stomach fluid and kidney essence flow upwards, just as "*Lianquan* and *Yuying* are the passages of thin fluid and thick fluid" recorded in the book *The Spiritual Pivot-Discussion on Distension*. Therefore, the amount of body fluid can be reflected on the tongue. The form, texture and color of the tongue are related to the sufficiency and insufficiency as well as the movement of qi and blood whereas the moist and dryness of the tongue fur and tongue body, to the amount of body fluid.

三、舌面与脏腑的对应关系
3. Correspondence of the tongue to the viscera

据古代医籍记载，脏腑的病变反映于舌面，有一定的分布规律，其中比较一致的说法是：舌尖多反映上焦心肺的病变；舌中多反映中焦脾胃的病变；舌根多反映下焦肾的病变；舌两侧多反映肝胆的病变（图 1.3.3.1）。

According to ancient medical literature, the viscera's disease is reflected on the surface of the tongue with a certain regularity of distribution. Namely, the tongue tip reflects the pathological changes of the heart and lungs; the center, the spleen and stomach; the root, the kidney; and the bilateral margins, the liver and gallbladder（Fig. 1.3.3.1）.

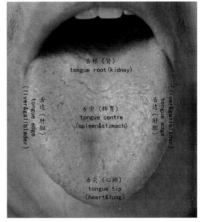

图 1.3.3.1
Fig. 1.3.3.1

总之，舌体虽小，但由于它与脏腑经络气血津液的联系紧密，故能客观、灵敏地反映它们的生理功能和病理变化。正如《伤寒指掌·察舌辨症法》所说："病之经络、脏腑、营卫、气血、表里、阴阳、寒热、虚实，毕形于舌。"

In conclusion, although small, the tongue is closely related to the viscera, meridians, qi, blood and fluid. So it can objectively and sensitively reflect its physiological functions and pathological changes. As stated in the book *A Handbook on Cold Damage-Syndrome Differentiation by Tongue Diagnosis*, "all the aspects of a disease can be exhibited on the tongue, including its location in meridians or viscera, nutrient or defense aspect, qi or blood, and its nature of exogenous or interior, yin or yang, cold or heat, deficiency or excess."

第四节　舌诊的临床意义

Section 4　Clinical Significance of the Tongue Diagnosis

　　舌象的变化能较客观准确地反映病情，可作为诊断疾病和辨证、立法、处方、用药的重要依据，对分析疾病的转归、预后都具有重要意义。

The changes of tongue manifestation objectively and exactly reflect the state of an illness. Therefore, they can be regarded as an important basis for disease diagnosis, syndrome differentiation, therapeutic principle, prescription and medication. It is of great significance for the analysis of diseases prognosis.

一、判断邪正盛衰

1. To judge the exuberance or debilitation of the vital-qi and the pathogenic-qi

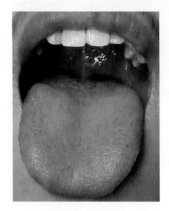

图 1.4.1.1
Fig. 1.4.1.1

　　邪气与正气之盛衰，可在舌象方面反映出来。舌体淡红，柔软灵活，苔薄白而润，说明正气充足，气血运行正常，津液末伤（图 1.4.1.1）；舌色淡白，是气血两虚（图 1.4.1.2）；舌干苔燥，是津液已伤（图 1.4.1.3）；舌苔有根，是胃气充足（图 1.4.1.4）；舌苔厚则为邪气盛（图 1.4.1.5）；舌苔无根或光剥无苔，是胃气衰败（图 1.4.1.6a，图 1.4.1.6b）。

The exuberance or debilitation of the healthy-qi and the pathogenic-qi can be shown in tongue. The soft and flexible tongue in pink color with thin, white and moist fur indicated sufficient vital-qi, the normal moving of qi and blood and the uninjured body fluid (Fig.1.4.1.1). The tongue in white color usually was resulted from the deficiency of both qi and blood (Fig.1.4.1.2). The dry tongue and fur was resulted from the impairment of body fluid (Fig.1.4.1.3). The rooted fur means sufficient stomach-qi (Fig.1.4.1.4). The thick fur suggested flourishing pathogenic-qi (Fig.1.4.1.5). While the non-rooted or whole exfoliated fur is usually caused by the declined stomach-qi (Fig.1.4.1.6a, Fig.1.4.1.6b).

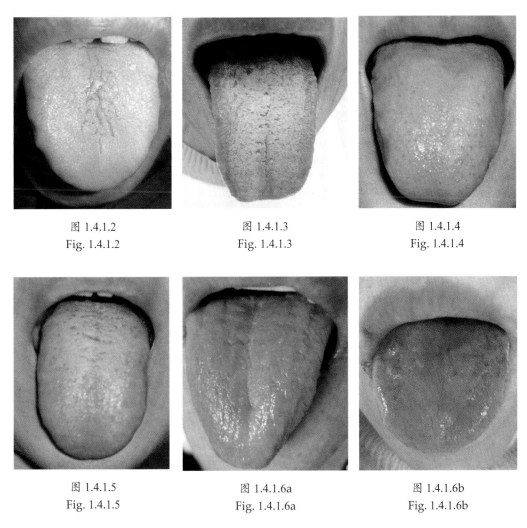

图 1.4.1.2
Fig. 1.4.1.2

图 1.4.1.3
Fig. 1.4.1.3

图 1.4.1.4
Fig. 1.4.1.4

图 1.4.1.5
Fig. 1.4.1.5

图 1.4.1.6a
Fig. 1.4.1.6a

图 1.4.1.6b
Fig. 1.4.1.6b

二、区别病邪性质

2. To distinguish the nature of disease pathogen

不同性质的邪气致病，在舌象上会反映出不同的变化。一般而言，外感风寒，苔多薄白（图 1.4.2.1）；外感风热，苔多薄黄（图 1.4.2.2）；寒湿为病，多舌胖苔腻（图 1.4.2.3）；燥邪为患，多舌红苔干（图 1.4.2.4）；火热内盛，多舌红苔黄燥（图 1.4.2.5）；痰浊内阻，苔多黏腻（图 1.4.2.6）；水饮停聚，苔多水滑（图 1.4.2.7）；食滞内停，苔多粗腐（图 1.4.2.8）；瘀血者，舌多见紫暗斑点（图 1.4.2.9）。

Pathogenic factors of different natures will make different changes in tongue. In general speaking, the thin and white fur mostly results from exogenous wind-cold (Fig.1.4.2.1). While thin and yellow fur often results from exogenous wind-heat (Fig.1.4.2.2). The enlarged and fat tongue with greasy fur on the surface is usually due to the retention of cold-dampness (Fig.1.4.2.3). The tongue in red color with dry fur always is caused by the attack of dry evils (Fig.1.4.2.4). The interior flourishing fire-heat often results in red tongue and dries, yellow fur (Fig.1.4.2.5). The internal retention of phlegm-turbid usually leads to sticky and greasy fur (Fig.1.4.2.6). The slippery fur, with much fluid on the surface, is mostly caused by the retention of water-phlegm (Fig.1.4.2.7). The rough and putrid fur indicates the food-retention (Fig.1.4.2.8). Dark purple spots on the tongue body mostly result from the blood stasis (Fig.1.4.2.9).

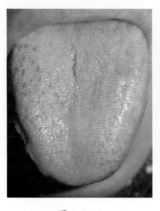 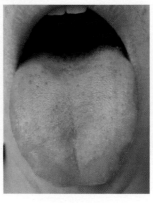 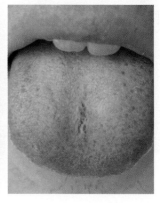

图 1.4.2.1   图 1.4.2.2   图 1.4.2.3

Fig. 1.4.2.1   Fig. 1.4.2.2   Fig. 1.4.2.3

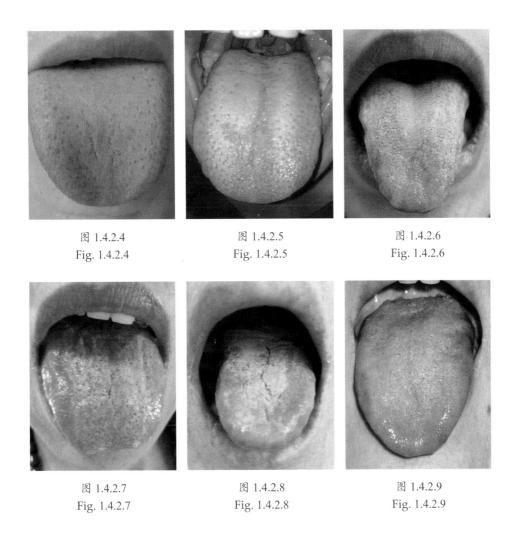

图 1.4.2.4　　　　　　　　　　图 1.4.2.5　　　　　　　　　　图 1.4.2.6
Fig. 1.4.2.4　　　　　　　　　Fig. 1.4.2.5　　　　　　　　　Fig. 1.4.2.6

图 1.4.2.7　　　　　　　　　　图 1.4.2.8　　　　　　　　　　图 1.4.2.9
Fig. 1.4.2.7　　　　　　　　　Fig. 1.4.2.8　　　　　　　　　Fig. 1.4.2.9

三、判别病位浅深

3. To detect the shallow or deep location of disease

病位的变化在舌象上也有相应的表现。大体而言，病邪轻浅，多见舌苔变化，而病情深重可见舌质、舌苔同时变化。如外感病中，苔薄白是疾病初起，病情轻浅（图 1.4.3.1）；苔黄厚，舌质红为病邪入里，病情较重，主气分热盛（图 1.4.3.2）；邪入营分，可见舌绛（图 1.4.3.3）；邪入血分，可见舌质深绛或紫暗，苔少或无苔（图 1.4.3.4）。以上说明不同的舌象提示病位浅深不同。

The changes of the location of disease can be reflected by tongue accordingly. In general, the light and shallow disease may cause the changes of tongue fur, while the deep and severe disease may result in the changes of tongue fur and texture at the same time. For example, the thin white fur suggests that the disease is in its initial stage, the disease was located in shallow part and it was an exterior syndrome (Fig.1.4.3.1). But the thick, yellow fur and red tongue suggested that the disease was severe, and there is excessive heat in the qi phase, it was an interior syndrome (Fig.1.4.3.2). The crimson tongue indicated that the evils already entered into the ying phase (Fig.1.4.3.3). The deep crimson or dark purple tongue with little fur or without any fur meant the evils into the blood phase (Fig.1.4.3.4). All of the above shown that the shallow or deep location of disease can be reflected by different tongue.

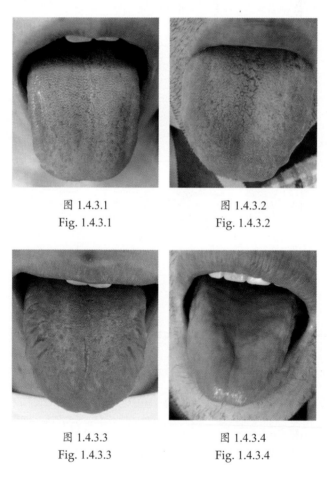

图 1.4.3.1
Fig. 1.4.3.1

图 1.4.3.2
Fig. 1.4.3.2

图 1.4.3.3
Fig. 1.4.3.3

图 1.4.3.4
Fig. 1.4.3.4

四、推断病势进退

4. To infer the tendency of disease

通过对舌象的动态观察，可测知疾病发展的进退趋势。从舌苔上看，若苔色由白转黄（图 1.4.4.1a，图 1.4.4.1b），由黄转为灰黑（图 1.4.4.2a，图 1.4.4.2b），苔质由薄转厚（图 1.4.4.3a，图 1.4.4.3b），由润转燥（图 1.4.4.4a，图 1.4.4.4b），多为病邪由表入里，由轻变重，由寒化热，邪热内盛，津液耗伤，为病势发展。反之，若舌苔由厚变薄（图 1.4.4.5a，图 1.4.4.5b），由黄转白（图 1.4.4.6a，图 1.4.4.6b），由燥转润（图 1.4.4.7a，图 1.4.4.7b），为病邪渐退，津液复生，病情向好的方向转变。从舌质上看，舌色由红转为绛或舌面有芒刺、裂纹（图 1.4.4.8a，图 1.4.4.8b），是邪热内入营血，有伤阴、血瘀之势；若淡红舌转淡白、淡紫湿润，舌体胖嫩有齿痕（图 1.4.4.9a，图 1.4.4.9b）为阳气受伤，阴寒内盛，病邪由表入里，由轻转重，病情由单纯变为复杂，为病进。

The changes of tongue usually followed the changes of genuine qi and evils, and disease location, so we can infer the development and tendency of the disease by observing the changes of the tongue. For example, if the fur color changes from white to yellow(Fig.1.4.4.1a, Fig.1.4.4.1b), or from yellow to gray-black (Fig.1.4.4.2a, Fig.1.4.4.2b), the fur texture changes from thin to thick (Fig.1.4.4.3a, Fig.1.4.4.3b), or from moist to dry (Fig.1.4.4.4a, Fig.1.4.4.4b), usually suggest the transferring of evils from exterior to interior, or from light to severe, or from cold to heat. These changes resulted in the impairment and exhaustion of body fluid by the internal flourishing heat evils. It shows the deterioration of disease. On the contrary, if the fur color changes from yellow to white (Fig.1.4.4.5a, Fig.1.4.4.5b), or the fur texture from thick to thin (Fig.1.4.4.6a, Fig.1.4.4.6b), or from dry to moist (Fig.1.4.4.7a, Fig.1.4.4.7b), suggest the slow withdrawal of evils and the production of new body fluid. It means the retreating of disease. If the tongue color turns from red to purple, or there being prickles and fissure on the tongue surface (Fig.1.4.48a, Fig.1.4.4.8b), it suggests that the heat evils have entered into the ying and blood phase and have tendency to injure yin and resulted in blood stasis. If the tongue color turns from pink to pale, or pale purple, or there being teeth-prints on the margin of the fat, tender tongue body (Fig.1.4.4.9a, Fig.1.4.4.9b), it is from the injured yang and the internal flourishing cold. It is a sign of that the evils has entered into the interior from the exterior and disease deteriorating.

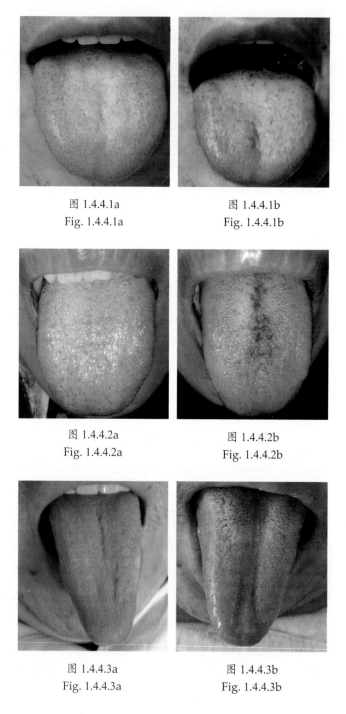

图 1.4.4.1a
Fig. 1.4.4.1a

图 1.4.4.1b
Fig. 1.4.4.1b

图 1.4.4.2a
Fig. 1.4.4.2a

图 1.4.4.2b
Fig. 1.4.4.2b

图 1.4.4.3a
Fig. 1.4.4.3a

图 1.4.4.3b
Fig. 1.4.4.3b

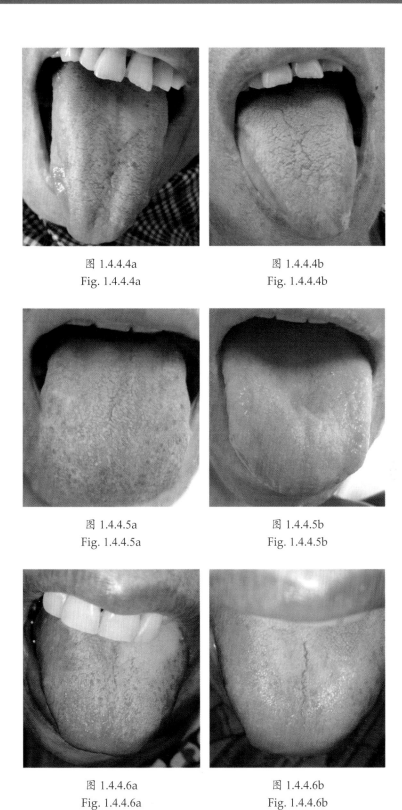

图 1.4.4.4a
Fig. 1.4.4.4a

图 1.4.4.4b
Fig. 1.4.4.4b

图 1.4.4.5a
Fig. 1.4.4.5a

图 1.4.4.5b
Fig. 1.4.4.5b

图 1.4.4.6a
Fig. 1.4.4.6a

图 1.4.4.6b
Fig. 1.4.4.6b

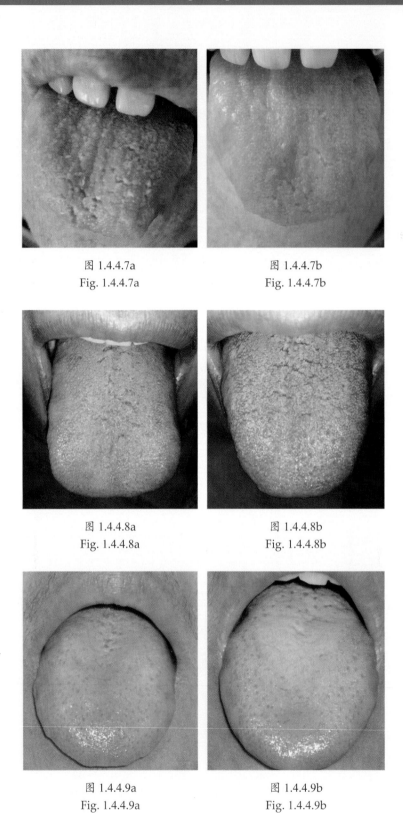

图 1.4.4.7a
Fig. 1.4.4.7a

图 1.4.4.7b
Fig. 1.4.4.7b

图 1.4.4.8a
Fig. 1.4.4.8a

图 1.4.4.8b
Fig. 1.4.4.8b

图 1.4.4.9a
Fig. 1.4.4.9a

图 1.4.4.9b
Fig. 1.4.4.9b

五、估计病情预后

5. To estimate the prognosis of disease

舌荣有神, 舌面有苔, 舌态正常者 (图 1.5.1.1), 为邪气未盛, 正气未伤, 胃气未败, 预后较好; 舌质枯晦, 舌苔无根, 舌态异常者 (图 1.5.1.2), 为正气亏虚, 胃气衰败, 病情多凶险。

If the tongue shows the vigor, fur on the surface of the tongue and the flexible movement of the tongue (Fig.1.5.1.1), it suggests that the evils is not flourishing, the vital-qi is not injured and the stomach-qi is not exhausted. It shows a good prognosis. The withering tongue texture with non-rooted fur and inflexible tongue indicates the deficiency of vital-qi and the exhaustion of stomach-qi (Fig.1.5.1.2). It suggests the deterioration of the disease.

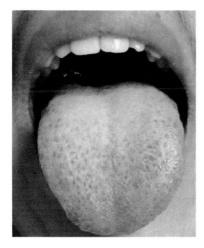
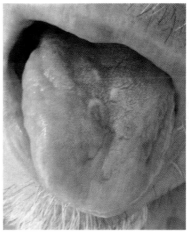

图 1.5.1.1   图 1.5.1.2
Fig. 1.5.1.1   Fig. 1.5.1.2

第二章 舌诊基础研究

Chapter 2　Basic Research of the Tongue Diagnosis

舌诊是通过诊察舌质和舌苔的变化，了解机体生理功能和病理变化的诊察方法。舌质是指舌的肌肉和脉络组织，舌苔是指舌面上附着的苔状物。

Looking at the tongue is a diagnostic method, Through observation of the tongue proper and tongue coating, physicians know both the physiological and pathological conditions of patients. The tongue body refers to the muscles and blood vessels of the tongue , tongue coating is a layer of moss-like matter spreading on the surface of tongue.

第一节　诊舌质

Section 1　Inspection of Tongue Texture

一、舌神

1.Tongue vitality (Spirit)

（一）有神（荣舌）

1.1　Full vitality（Luxuriant tongue）

［舌象特征］舌质红润，活动自如（图 2.1.1.1）。

［Characteristics of the tongue］The tongue is ruddy, and its movement is flexible（Fig 2.1.1.1）.

［临床意义］气血充沛、正常舌象或病情轻浅，预后良好。

［Clinical significance］It suggests plentiful qi and Blood. It is normal tongue characteristic or presents with mild illnesses. The prognosis are good.

［机理分析］《辨舌指南·辨舌之神气》："荣者，有光彩也，凡病皆吉；荣润则津足。荣者谓有神······凡舌质有光有体，无论黄、白、灰、黑，刮之而里面红润，神气荣华者，诸病皆吉。"

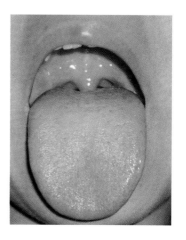

图 2.1.1.1
Fig. 2.1.1.1

［Mechanism analysis］*Guide to Tongue Diagnosis-Differentiation of the Tongue Vitality* said: "The flourish of tongue means the tongue has luster and the prognosis is good. The flourish of tongue refers to enough fluid in it. The flourish means full of vitality... If the tongue shows red, moist and vigorous, no matter the color of tongue fur is yellow, white or black, the prognosis is good."

（二）无神（枯舌）

1.2 Lacking of vitality（Withered tongue）

［舌象特征］舌质晦暗干枯，活动不灵活（图 2.1.1.2）。

［Characteristics of the tongue］The tongue lacking of vitality refers to dark and dry tongue texture and tongue body with sluggish movement (Fig 2.1.1.2).

［临床意义］脏腑气血亏虚，病情较重或预后不良。

［Clinical significance］It suggests exhausting of *zang-fu* qi and blood, and the prognosis is bad in this condition.

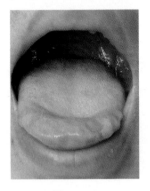

图 2.1.1.2
Fig. 2.1.1.2

［机理分析］《辨舌指南·辨舌之神气》曰："枯者，无精神也，凡病皆凶；干枯则津乏。枯者谓无神……若舌质无光无体，不拘有苔无苔，视之里面枯晦，神气全无者，诸病皆凶。"

［Mechanism analysis］*Guide to Tongue Diagnosis-Differentiation of the Tongue Vitality* said: "The withering is out of vitality and the prognosis is bad. The withering suggests the lacking of blood of the body that will be dying... If the condition is dark and dry, no matter there is fur or not, the prognosis is very bad."

二、舌色

2. Tongue color

（一）淡红舌

2.1 Pink tongue

［舌象特征］舌体颜色淡红润泽，不浅不深，红淡适中（图 2.1.2.1a）。

［Characteristics of the tongue］The tongue body is pink and lustrous. The normal condition is neither too light nor too deep pink color of whole tongue body (Fig 2.1.2.1a).

［临床意义］淡红舌为正常舌象，反映心血充足，胃气旺盛。其是气血调和的征象，常见于健康人，疾病时见之属病轻。

［Clinical significance］Pink is the normal color of tongue body. It suggests sufficient heart blood and vigorous stomach qi. It means reconciliation of qi and blood, which is often seen in healthy people, or sign of a mild case when it is seen in patients.

[**机理分析**] 淡红舌主要反映心血充足、胃气健旺的生理状态。其是气血调和的征象。故《舌胎统志•淡红舌》说："舌色淡红，平人之候……红者心之气，淡者胃之气。"《舌鉴辨正•红舌总论》亦说："全舌淡红，不浅不深者，平人也。"

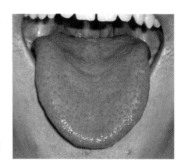

图 2.1.2.1a
Fig. 2.1.2.1a

[Mechanism analysis] Pink tongue suggests sufficient heart blood and vigorous stomach qi. It means reconciliation of qi and blood. *Records of Tongue fur-Light red Tongue* said, "The pink is normal color of the tongue body. The red tongue comes from heart qi and the pale comes from stomach qi." *Syndrome Differentiation on Tongue-red tongue refers* said: "Pink is the normal color of the tongue body, which is neither too light nor too deep, and usually can be seen from a healthy person."

外感病初期，舌色淡红，为外邪侵犯肌表，尚未侵及气血与脏腑，属病情轻浅（图 2.1.2.1b）；内伤杂病中见之，提示气血调和，多属病轻或疾病转愈之象（图 2.1.2.1c）。

A pink tongue in the early period of the exogenous diseases suggests that the disease is the exterior and not in qi, blood and *zang-fu*, and the state of illness was light (Fig. 2.1.2.1b). If it occurs in the case of internal injury, it indicates reconciliation of qi and blood, which is a sign of a mild case or recovery (Fig. 2.1.2.1c).

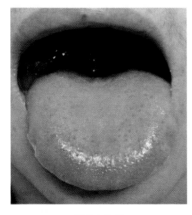

图 2.1.2.1b
Fig. 2.1.2.1b

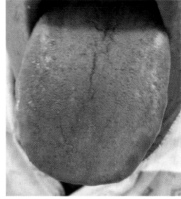

图 2.1.2.1c
Fig. 2.1.2.1c

（二）淡白舌

2.2　Pale tongue

［**舌象特征**］舌色比正常舌浅淡，白色偏多而红色偏少（图 2.1.2.2a）。

［Characteristics of the tongue］The tongue color is lighter than that of normal is known as pale tongue, which shows less red and much more white color (Fig.2.1.2.2a).

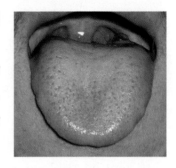

图 2.1.2.2a
Fig. 2.1.2.2a

［**临床意义**］主气血两虚、阳虚。

［Clinical significance］It is seen in cases of deficiency qi and blood, or yang.

［**机理分析**］气血亏虚，血不荣舌；阳气虚衰，运血无力，或阳虚内寒，经脉收引，气血不能上荣于舌。

［Mechanism analysis］It is due to decline of qi and blood, or yang deficiency. The deficient yang and qi fails to send blood up to the tongue, and the deficient blood fails to nourish the tongue, interior cold and contracture of the channels due to deficiency of yang failing to provide adequate blood to nourish the tongue.

舌色淡白而舌体瘦小（图 2.1.2.2 b），多为气血两虚，血不上荣；若舌色淡白，几无血色，干枯少津，则称为枯白舌（图 2.1.2.2c），多为阳虚不能运血，或脱血夺气，气血失充；若舌色淡白，舌体胖嫩，舌边有齿印，舌面湿润多津者（图 2.1.2.2d），多为阳虚水湿内停；若舌色淡白，舌面光滑无苔，则称为淡白光莹舌（图 2.1.2.2e），为脾胃之气衰败、气血衰败之候。

In general, the pale tongue with an emaciated body suggests the deficiency of both qi and blood and the deficient blood is failed to nourish the tongue (Fig.2.1.2.2b). While the pale tongue with less red color and fluid is named withered pale tongue (Fig.2.1.2.2c), suggests the deficiency yang which fails to carry blood, or the depletion of qi and blood which fails to nourish the tongue. The pale tongue with the fatter body and teeth-print and much fluid on fur implies the deficiency of yang and water-dampness detention (Fig.2.1.2.2d). While a pale slippery tongue without fur is called pale transparent tongue (Fig.2.1.2.2d), suggests the exhaustion of qi and blood, and extremely deficient qi of spleen and stomach.

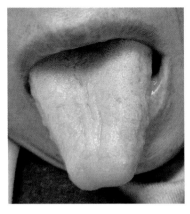

图 2.1.2.2b
Fig. 2.1.2.2b

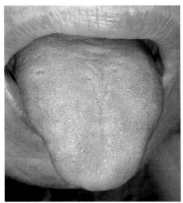

图 2.1.2.2c
Fig. 2.1.2.2c

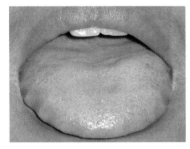

图 2.1.2.2d
Fig. 2.1.2.2d

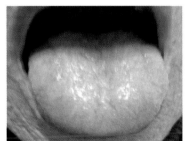

图 2.1.2.2e
Fig. 2.1.2.2e

（三）红舌

2.3　Red tongue

［**舌象特征**］舌色较淡红颜色为深，呈鲜红色（图 2.1.2.3a）。

［Characteristics of the tongue］The tongue is redder than normal or even brightly red (Fig. 2.1.2.3a).

［**临床意义**］主热证，包括实热和虚热。

［Clinical significance］It suggests internal heat. It indicates excess heat or internal heat form yin deficiency.

［**机理分析**］红舌乃热邪所致，血得热则血行加速，舌体脉络充盈而舌色变红。

［Mechanism analysis］The red tongue is caused by hot evil. Red tongue whose vessels are full of blood is caused by heat which speeds up the circulation of qi and blood.

舌边尖红（图 2.1.2.3b），多为外感风热表证初期；舌尖红赤破碎（图 2.1.2.3c），多为心火上炎；舌边红赤，多为肝胆有热（图 2.1.2.3d）；舌色红，舌尖有芒刺，舌面兼黄厚苔者（图 2.1.2.3e），多属实热证。舌色红舌体瘦小而干，舌面少苔或无苔，或有裂纹者（图 2.1.2.3f），多属虚热证。

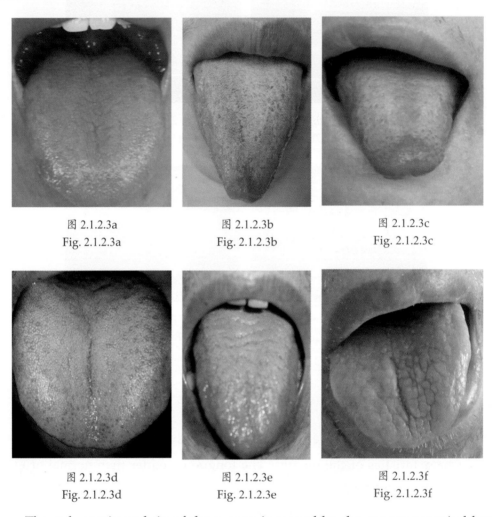

图 2.1.2.3a
Fig. 2.1.2.3a

图 2.1.2.3b
Fig. 2.1.2.3b

图 2.1.2.3c
Fig. 2.1.2.3c

图 2.1.2.3d
Fig. 2.1.2.3d

图 2.1.2.3e
Fig. 2.1.2.3e

图 2.1.2.3f
Fig. 2.1.2.3f

The red margin and tip of the tongue is caused by the exogenous wind-heat (Fig. 2.1.2.3b). When the tongue tip is red and ruptured, it dues to heart fire flaming up (Fig. 2.1.2.3c). The red tongue in bilateral margins dues to liver and gallbladder fire(Fig. 2.1.2.3d). The bright red tongue with rough and prickly fur or with thick and yellowish fur mostly suggests excess-heat syndrome (Fig. 2.1.2.3e). A withered red tongue and tongue body is thin, with less fur or without any fur or with crack on the body (Fig. 2.1.2.3f), which indicates a deficiency-heat syndrome.

（四）绛舌

2.4 Crimson Tongue

［舌象特征］舌色比红舌更深，或呈暗红色（图 2.1.2.4a ）。

［Characteristics of the tongue］The color is heavier and darker than red tongue or even dark red (Fig.2.1.2.4a).

［临床意义］主热盛。里热炽盛，阴虚火旺。

［Clinical significance］The tongue is often seen in the stage of extreme fever or indicates excessive heat or hyperactivity of fire from deficiency of yin.

［机理分析］绛舌多由红舌进一步发展而成，多因热入营血，耗伤营阴，血液浓缩或阴虚水涸，虚火上炎所致。舌绛在外感病中出现，为热邪侵入营血之征象，多见舌绛而干，或伴见芒刺（图 2.1.2.4b ）；在内伤病中出现，为阴液亏虚，虚火亢盛之候，多见舌绛少苔或无苔，或有裂纹（图 2.1.2.4c ）。若舌绛而光莹，为胃肾阴亏已竭（图 2.1.2.4d ）。

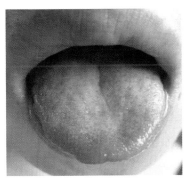
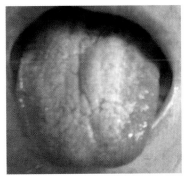

图 2.1.2.4a
Fig. 2.1.2.4a

图 2.1.2.4b
Fig. 2.1.2.4b

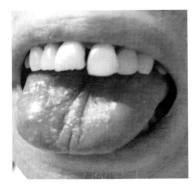
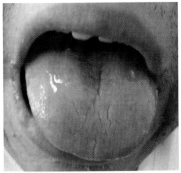

图 2.1.2.4c
Fig. 2.1.2.4c

图 2.1.2.4d
Fig. 2.1.2.4d

[Mechanism analysis] Crimson tongue comes from red tongue. It is resulted from upward invasion of asthenia heat. Because of deficiency of yin and exhaustion of fluid, or the exhaustion of yin and yin was hurt by the heat that results in blood concentrated. A dry crimson tongue, or with prickles, which can be seen in the exogenous diseased, suggests invasion into yin and blood by heat evil (Fig. 2.1.2.4b). A crimson tongue with less fur or no fur or with crack, which usually can be seen in the endogenous injury, suggests excessive asthenia heat resulting from deficiency of yin and fluid (Fig. 2.1.2.4c). A crimson with transparent fur results from exhaustion of yin of stomach and kidney (Fig. 2.1.2.4d).

（五）青紫舌

2.5 Bluish purple tongue

[舌象特征] 舌呈现青色或紫色者，为青紫舌（图 2.1.2.5a）；舌淡泛现青紫色，为淡紫舌（图 2.1.2.5b）；舌红而紫者，为紫红舌（图 2.1.2.5c）；舌绛而紫者为绛紫舌（图 2.1.2.5d）；舌现青紫色斑点，大小不等且不高于舌面者，为瘀点舌或瘀斑舌（图 2.1.2.5e）。

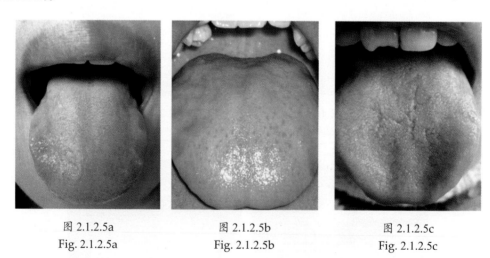

图 2.1.2.5a　　　　　　图 2.1.2.5b　　　　　　图 2.1.2.5c
Fig. 2.1.2.5a　　　　　　Fig. 2.1.2.5b　　　　　　Fig. 2.1.2.5c

[Characteristics of the tongue] The whole tongue which is bluish or purplish is called cyanotic tongue (Fig. 2.1.2.5a). The tongue which is pale and present with blue-purple (Fig. 2.1.2.5b) is called light purple tongue. The tongue which is red and purple is called purplish red tongue (Fig. 2.1.2.5c). The tongue which is crimson and purple is called deep purple tongue (Fig. 2.1.2.5d). When bluish purple spots appear on a part the tongue, and they are of different size and not above the surface. These tongue are called spotted or ecchymosis tongue (Fig. 2.1.2.5e).

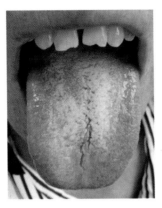

图 2.1.2.5d
Fig. 2.1.2.5d

图 2.1.2.5e
Fig. 2.1.2.5e

［临床意义］主气血运行不畅，血瘀。

［Clinical significance］It indicates unsmooth movement of qi and blood, and blood stasis.

［机理分析］舌淡紫或青紫湿润主寒证（图 2.1.2.5f）；舌色淡紫，或紫暗而湿润，多为阳虚寒盛，气血运行不畅之证（图 2.1.2.5g）；舌红紫干枯少津主热证（图 2.1.2.5h）；舌色绛紫，干枯少津，多为火热炽盛，营阴受损之证（图 2.1.2.5i）；舌色青紫，多为寒凝气滞，血液瘀阻之证，也可见于先天性心脏病，或药物、食物中毒等病证。

［Mechanism analysis］A pale or darken moist purple tongue suggests coldness (Fig.2.1.2.5f). The pale or darken moist purple tongue mostly results from the stagnation of qi and blood caused by yang deficiency which fails to warm and push them in movement (Fig.2.1.2.5g). While a withered red purple with less fluid suggests heat syndromes (Fig.2.1.2.5h). The withered crimson purple tongue always dues to injury of nutrient-yin caused by excessive heat (Fig.2.1.2.5i). When the tongue body is light blue and purple, it is called bluish purple tongue. It dues to coagulated blood and stagnated qi by the coldness, congenital heart diseases, and the syndromes caused by toxin of food and drugs poisoning.

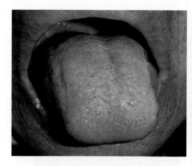

图 2.1.2.5f
Fig. 2.1.2.5f

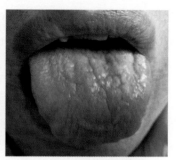

图 2.1.2.5g
Fig. 2.1.2.5g

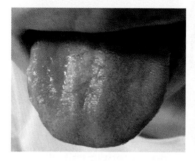

图 2.1.2.5h
Fig. 2.1.2.5h

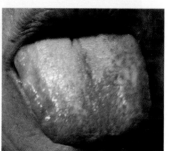

图 2.1.2.5i
Fig. 2.1.2.5i

三、舌形

3.Tongue shape

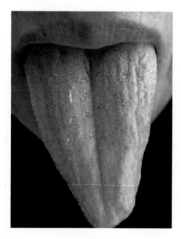

图 2.1.3.1a
Fig. 2.1.3.1a

（一）老、嫩舌

3.1　Tough and tender tongue

［**舌象特征**］舌质纹理粗糙,坚不柔软,舌色较暗者,为苍老舌（图 2.1.3.1a）；舌质纹理细腻，浮胖娇嫩，舌色较淡者，为娇嫩舌（图 2.1.3.1b）。

［Characteristics of the Tongue］Striated of tongue are rough and sturdy and the color of tongue is dark. It was also called the tough tongue (Fig.2.1.3.1a). Striated of tongue are delicate, fine and smooth, and the color of the tongue is light. It was called the tender tongue (Fig.2.1.3.1b).

［临床意义］老舌多见于实证，嫩舌多见于虚证。

［Clinical significance］The old tongue is more often seen in the excess syndromes, and the tender tongue is more common in the deficiency syndrome.

［机理分析］《辨舌指南》说："凡舌质坚敛而苍老，不拘苔色黄白灰黑，病多属实。舌质浮胖娇嫩，不拘苔色灰黑黄白，病多属虚。"实邪亢盛而正气未衰，邪正交争，则邪气壅滞于舌上，故见舌质苍老。气血亏虚或阳气不足，脉络不充，运血不力，以致舌质娇嫩。

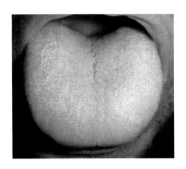

图 2.1.3.1b
Fig. 2.1.3.1b

［Mechanism analysis］*Guide to Tongue Diagnosis* said: "A rough and sturdy tongue, no matter with yellowish, gray or black fur, usually indicated excess syndrome. A tender tongue, no matter with gray, black yellowish or white fur, mostly indicated deficiency syndromes." The rough tongue resulted from excessive evil congesting in the body, with which underlining genuine-qi fight, and the stagnation in the upper-jiao because of the evil. The tender tongue resulted from deficient qi and blood falling to full channels and collateral in the tongue, or deficient yang failing to carry blood to nourish the tongue body.

（二）胖、瘦舌

3.2　Enlarged and thin tongue

［舌象特征］舌体较正常舌大而厚，伸舌满口，称为胖大舌（图 2.1.3.2a）；舌体肿大，伸舌盈口满嘴，甚则不能回缩，称为胖胀舌（图 2.1.3.2b）；舌体较正常瘦小而薄，则为瘦薄舌（图 2.1.3.2c）。

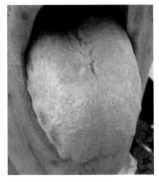 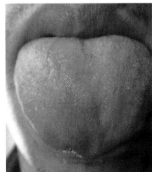 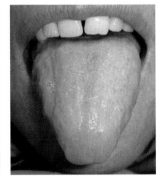

图 2.1.3.2a　　　　　　图 2.1.3.2b　　　　　　图 2.1.3.2c
Fig. 2.1.3.2a　　　　　　Fig. 2.1.3.2b　　　　　　Fig. 2.1.3.2c

［Characteristics of the Tongue］The enlarged and swollen tongue body, even filling up mouth, was called a swollen tongue (Fig.2.1.3.2a). The tongue body large in size, even filling up the whole mouth, or even failing to shrink back, was called a fat swollen tongue (Fig.2.1.3.2b). A tongue smaller and thinner than normal in size was called thin tongue (Fig. 2.1.3.2c).

［**临床意义**］胖大舌多主痰湿热毒或水湿内停。瘦薄舌多主气血两虚或阴虚火旺。

［Clinical significance］A big fat tongue suggests phlegm dampness heat toxin or dampness retention. Thin tongue usually caused by the deficient qi and blood or hyperactivity of fire due to deficiency of yin.

［**机理分析**］舌淡胖大，舌面水滑，为脾肾阳虚，津液不化，水饮内停（图2.1.3.2d）；舌体红赤胖大，舌面有黄腻苔者，为脾胃湿热，或心胃热盛（图2.1.3.2e）；舌体绛紫肿大，为酒毒上冲，心火上炎（图2.3.3.5f）；舌青紫肿胀，为中毒血瘀（图2.1.3.2g）；舌体淡白瘦薄，为气血两虚（图2.1.3.2h）；舌体嫩红瘦薄，为心阴不足（图2.1.3.2i）；舌体红绛瘦薄，为阴虚火旺（图2.1.3.2j）。

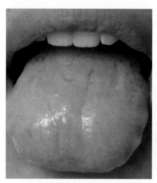 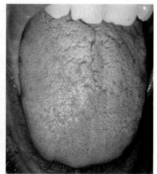

图 2.1.3.2d　　　　　图 2.1.3.2e
Fig. 2.1.3.2d　　　　　Fig. 2.1.3.2e

［Mechanism analysis］The pale and puffy tongue with moist fur is usually attributed to insufficiency of spleen-yang and kidney-yang and accumulation of the phlegm-damp (Fig. 2.1.3.2d). The red and corpulent tongue with yellow and greasy fur to damp-heat in the spleen and stomach, or excessive heat in the heart and stomach (Fig. 2.1.3.2e). The purplish and swollen tongue, to upward attack of fire in the heart with alcoholic toxicity (Fig. 2.1.3.2f). The puffy, bluish-purple and lusterless tongue, accompanying with blue lip, to stagnation of blood frequently seen in poisoning (Fig. 2.1.3.2g). The pale thin tongue is usually due to qi and blood deficiency (Fig. 2.1.3.2h). The tender red thin tongue is usually due to insufficient yin in the heart (Fig. 2.1.3.2i). The dry thin tongue in red or crimson is often due to fire flaring in yin deficiency (Fig. 2.1.3.2j).

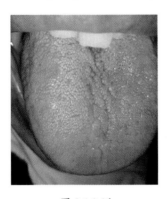 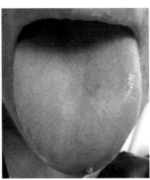 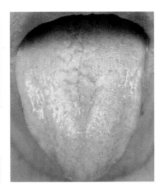

图 2.1.3.2f   图 2.1.3.2g   图 2.1.3.2h
Fig. 2.1.3.2f   Fig. 2.1.3.2g   Fig. 2.1.3.2h

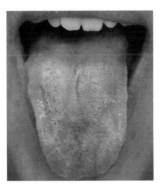 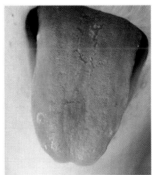

图 2.1.3.2i   图 2.1.3.2j
Fig. 2.1.3.2i   Fig. 2.1.3.2j

（三）齿痕舌

3.3 Teeth-marked tongue

［**舌象特征**］舌体边缘有牙齿压迫的痕迹（图 2.1.3.3a）。

［Characteristics of the Tongue］The tongue with tooth prints at its borders was known as teeth-printed tongue (Fig.2.1.3.3a).

［**临床意义**］主脾虚证，或水湿内盛证。

［Clinical significance］It mostly resulted from spleen deficiency and excessive dampness.

［**机理分析**］齿痕舌多与胖大舌同见，因舌体胖大而受牙齿挤压所致。

舌淡胖大而有齿痕者（图 2.1.3.3b），多属阳虚寒湿内盛，或脾气虚；若舌红而肿胀有齿痕者（图 2.1.3.3c），则为湿热痰浊内壅。

［Mechanism analysis］The teeth-marked tongue is often seen in swollen tongue which is pressed by teeth.

The pale and moist tongue with tooth prints at its borders usually suggests an excess of cold of cold-dampness (Fig.2.1.3.3b). Whereas the red and swollen tongue filling up the mouth with tooth marks on its margin (Fig.2.1.3.3c), suggest the stagnation of internal damp-heat and phlegm.

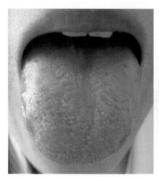 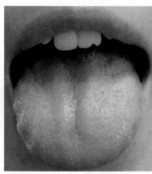 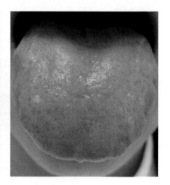

| 图 2.1.3.3a | 图 2.1.3.3b | 图 2.1.3.3c |
| Fig 2.1.3.3a | Fig. 2.1.3.3b | Fig. 2.1.3.3c |

（四）点、刺舌

3.4　Pointed and pricked tongue

［**舌象特征**］点，是指蕈状乳头增大，数目增多，乳头充血水肿。其中大者称星，称红星舌（图 2.1.3.4a）；小者称点，称红点舌（图 2.1.3.4b）。刺，是指蕈状乳头增大、高突，并形成尖锋，形如芒刺，模之棘手，称为芒刺舌（图 2.1.3.4c）。

［Characteristics of the tongue］Point refers to mushroom papillae on the surface of the tongue congestion and edema, the papillae become large and more, while the big one is named as star (Fig.2.1.3.4a), and the small one is called point (Fig.2.1.3.4b). The hyperplasic lingual papillae, protruding like the thorns and causing a prickly sensation when they are palpated with finger are known as the prickled tongue (Fig.2.1.3.4c).

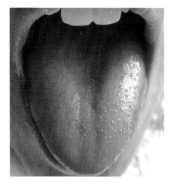
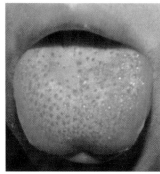
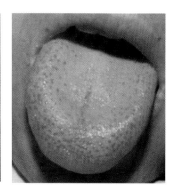

图 2.1.3.4a
Fig. 2.1.3.4a

图 2.1.3.4b
Fig. 2.1.3.4b

图 2.1.3.4c
Fig. 2.1.3.4c

［临床意义］主脏腑阳热亢盛或血分热盛。

［Clinical significance］It suggests exuberant yang heat in the *zang-fu* organs or excessive heat in blood.

［机理分析］点刺舌多因邪热亢盛、脏腑热极、瘟毒入血、湿热蕴于血分所致。一般点刺愈多，邪热愈甚。

舌尖有点刺（图 2.1.3.4d），多提示心火旺盛；舌边有点刺（图 2.1.3.4e），多为肝胆有热；舌中有点刺（图 2.1.3.4f），多属胃肠热盛。

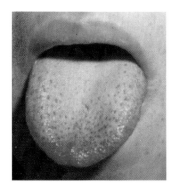
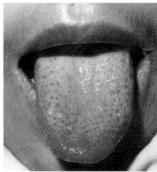
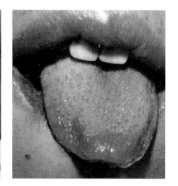

图 2.1.3.4d
Fig. 2.1.3.4d

图 2.1.3.4e
Fig. 2.1.3.4e

图 2.1.3.4f
Fig. 2.1.3.4f

［Mechanism analysis］They are mostly caused by excessive heat evils, extreme heat in *zang-fu*, or the attack into the blood by pestilence poisoning or stagnation of damp-heat in blood. The more exorbitant the heat evils are, the more and larger the awn-prickles are.

Prickles on tongue tip are due to flaring fire in the heart (Fig.2.1.3.4d). Prickles on the sides of tongue are due to heat in the liver and gallbladder (Fig.2.1.3.4e).

Prickles on middle tongue are due to heat in the stomach and intestines(Fig.2.1.3.4f).

（五）裂纹舌

3.5 Fissured tongue

[舌象特征]舌面上呈现多少不等、深浅不一、形状各异的裂沟或皱纹，沟裂中无舌苔覆盖，称为裂纹舌（图 2.1.3.5a ）。

[Characteristics of the tongue]If there are cracks in different size, depth, and shape on tongue without any fur cover, it is called a crack tongue (Fig.2.1.3.5a).

[临床意义]多因血虚失养、热灼津伤或阴液亏虚所致。

[Clinical significance]It is caused by deficient blood with malnutrition, fluid injury, or deficient blood yin resulted from excessive heat.

[机理分析]舌色淡白而有裂纹或裂沟者（图 2.1.3.5b ），为血虚之候；舌红绛而有裂纹者（图 2.1.3.5c ），多因邪热内盛，热盛伤津，阴津耗伤。

[Mechanism analysis]The pale tongue with fissures (Fig.2.1.3.5b), suggests deficiency of blood. The dark red tongue with fissures (Fig.2.1.3.5c), means the excessive heat in *zang-fu* which consume the fluid.

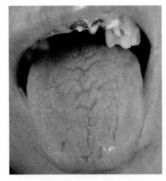
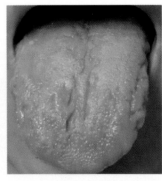
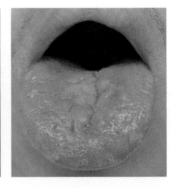

图 2.1.3.5a   图 2.1.3.5b   图 2.1.3.5c
Fig. 2.1.3.5a   Fig. 2.1.3.5b   Fig. 2.1.3.5c

四、舌态

4. Tongue motility

（一）痿软舌

4.1　Flaccid tongue

［舌象特征］舌体软弱无力，不能随意伸缩回旋（图 2.1.4.1a ）。

［Characteristics of the Tongue］If the tongue is weak and unable to protrude and curl, it is called flaccid tongue (Fig. 2.1.4.1a).

［临床意义］多为气血两虚、热灼阴液耗损致舌体筋脉失养所致。

［Clinical significance］Resulted mostly from the protracted deficiency of qi and blood or consumption of yin fluid due to excessive heat.

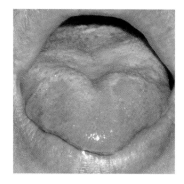

图 2.1.4.1a
Fig. 2.1.4.1a

［机理分析］舌体痿软舌色淡白者，为气血两虚，久病舌体失养（图 2.1.4.1b ）；若舌体痿软而舌红苔黄者，是热灼津伤（图 2.1.4.1c ）；舌体痿软而舌绛光滑者，外感病属热极伤阴，内伤病属阴虚火旺（图 2.1.4.1d ）。

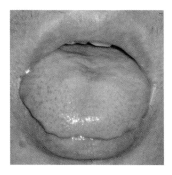

图 2.1.4.1b
Fig. 2.1.4.1b

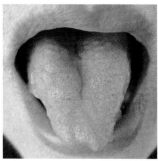

图 2.1.4.1c
Fig. 2.1.4.1c

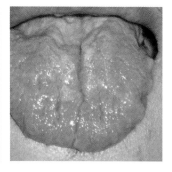

图 2.1.4.1d
Fig. 2.1.4.1d

［Mechanism analysis］The flaccid tongue in pale color in chronic diseases is usually due to deficiency of both qi and blood, because of malnutrition of muscles, tendons and vessels (Fig. 2.1.4.1b). The flaccid tongue in red color with yellow fur is due to injury of body fluid consumed by excessive heat (Fig. 2.1.4.1c). The smooth and flaccid tongue in crimson color usually belongs to impairment of yin, because of extremely intense pathogenic heat in exogenous diseases, or the flaring fire and deficient yin in internal diseases (Fig. 2.1.4.1d).

（二）强硬舌

4.2 Stiff tongue

［舌象特征］舌体不能转动，板硬强直，以致伸缩不利，舌失柔和（图 2.1.4.2a）。

［Characteristics of the Tongue］It is an inflexible tongue with difficulty in moving or inability of turning (Fig.2.1.4.2a).

［临床意义］多为热入心包，或高热津伤（图 2.1.4.2b），或风痰阻络（图 2.1.4.2c）。

［Clinical significance］It mostly results from an attack of the pericardium caused by excessive heat, or heat impairment of body fluid because of extremely intense pathogenic heat (Fig.2.1.4.2b) or wind-phlegm obstructing the meridians in tongue (Fig.2.1.4.2c).

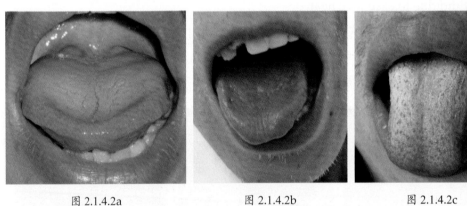

图 2.1.4.2a
Fig. 2.1.4.2a

图 2.1.4.2b
Fig. 2.1.4.2b

图 2.1.4.2c
Fig. 2.1.4.2c

［机理分析］《备急千金要方》说："舌强不能言，病在脏腑。"《辨舌指南》指出："凡红舌强硬，为脏腑实热已极。"

［Mechanism analysis］*Important Formulas Worth a Thousand Gold Pieces* said: "a patient can't speak with stiff tongue, it suggested the diseases lie in *zang-fu*." And the *Guide to Tongue Diagnosis* had referred: "all the stiff tongue in red color is due to extreme excessive heat in *zang-fu*."

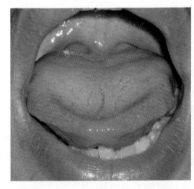 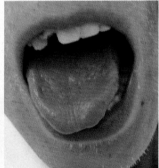 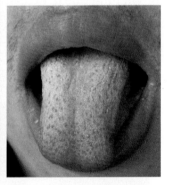

syndromes, the light or shallow interior syndromes, or the interior cold resulting from deficient yang (Fig.2.2.2.1d). The thin, white and slippery fur is mostly due to the exterior cold-dampness, or the internal retention of water-dampness caused by deficient spleen-yang and kidney-yang (Fig.2.2.2.1e). The thin, white and dry fur is usually due to the exterior wind-heat (Fig.2.2.2.1f). The white, thick and greasy fur often resulted from the internal retention of turbid dampness and phlegm caused by uninspired middle-yang, or the retention of food in the stomach and intestines (Fig.2.2.2.1g). The thick, white and dry fur indicated the internal accumulation of phlegm and damp-heat (Fig.2.2.2.1h). The white fur spreading over the tongue like the heaped powder, but not being dry while palpated is called the powder-like fur, as a result of the combination of the filthy and turbid dampness with the heat toxin (Fig.2.2.2.1i). It is often seen in pestilence and abscess of internal organs. The white and dry fur like sand, being rough while palpated, suggests the damaged body fluid by dry-heat and the exhaustion of yin-fluid (Fig.2.2.2.1j).

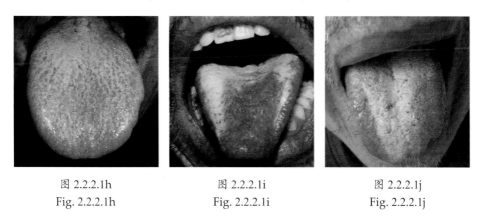

图 2.2.2.1h 图 2.2.2.1i 图 2.2.2.1j
Fig. 2.2.2.1h Fig. 2.2.2.1i Fig. 2.2.2.1j

（二）黄苔

2.2　Yellow fur

［**舌象特征**］舌面上所附着的苔垢呈现黄色，称为黄苔（图 2.2.2.2a）。据苔黄的程度，有淡黄、深黄和焦黄之分（图 2.2.2.2b，图 2.2.2.2c，图 2.2.2.2d）。

［Characteristics of the Tongue］The fur being adhered to the surface of the tongue in yellow color called yellow fur (Fig.2.2.2.2a). It can be divided into light yellow, heavy yellow and brown yellow fur (Fig.2.2.2.2b, Fig.2.2.2.2c, Fig.2.2.2.2d).

［**临床意义**］主热证、里证。

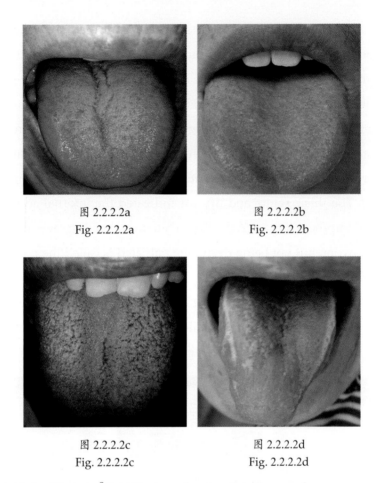

图 2.2.2.2a
Fig. 2.2.2.2a

图 2.2.2.2b
Fig. 2.2.2.2b

图 2.2.2.2c
Fig. 2.2.2.2c

图 2.2.2.2d
Fig. 2.2.2.2d

［Clinical significance］It indicates a heat or interior syndrome.

［**机理分析**］黄苔多因感受热邪或病邪入里化热，邪热熏灼于舌所致。

黄苔多为热邪熏灼于舌。黄苔色愈深，说明热邪愈甚。淡黄苔为热轻，深黄苔为热重，焦黄苔为热极。

［Mechanism analysis］The yellow fur mostly results from the invasion of heat evils, or the evil from the exterior into the interior producing heat and the heat evils stifling on the tongue. The deeper the yellow of the tongue fur, the more intense the pathogenic heat. The light yellow fur suggests shallow heat, while heave yellow fur indicates deep heat and brown yellow fur suggests extremely excessive heat.

舌苔由白转黄，或呈黄白相兼（图 2.2.2.2e），为外感表证处于化热入里，表里相兼阶段；苔色淡黄，苔质较薄者，为风热之邪犯表或风寒郁遏化热入里（图 2.2.2.2f）；苔色深黄，为里热夹湿，或痰饮化热，或食积热腐（图 2.2.2.2g）；苔色焦黄，为里热伤津，腑实燥结（图 2.2.2.2h）。

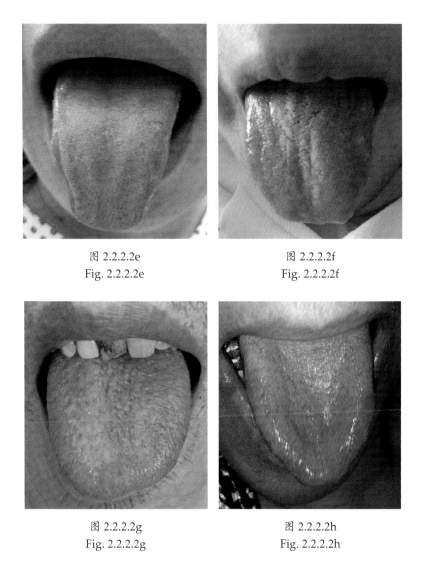

图 2.2.2.2e
Fig. 2.2.2.2e

图 2.2.2.2f
Fig. 2.2.2.2f

图 2.2.2.2g
Fig. 2.2.2.2g

图 2.2.2.2h
Fig. 2.2.2.2h

The change of tongue fur from white to yellow or to white-yellow (Fig. 2.2.2.2e) respectively suggests that the exterior syndrome of external contraction has transformed into heat and transmitted to the interior or to half-exterior and half-interior. Thin and light yellow fur indicates that pathogenic wind-heat invaded the exterior or depressed wind-cold has transformed into heat and transmitted to the interior (Fig. 2.2.2.2f). Deep yellow fur signifies internal heat complicated with dampness, or phlegm and fluid-retention transforming into heat, or food accumulation and heat putrefaction (Fig.2.2.2.2g). And scorched yellow fur hints internal heat consuming body fluid and excess syndrome of *fu*-organs with dry feces (Fig.2.2.2.2h).

苔淡黄而润滑多津者，称为黄滑苔（图 2.2.2.2i ），多为阳虚寒湿之体，痰饮聚久化热，或为气血亏虚，复感湿热之邪所致。黄苔而质腻者，称黄腻苔（图 2.2.2.2j ），主湿热或痰热内蕴，或为食积化腐。

The yellow slippery fur is named because the fur is moist, slippery, in light yellow color and with much fluid on the tongue surface (Fig. 2.2.2.2i). It mostly results from heat transformed from the long accumulated phlegm in patients with constitution of deficient yang and cold-dampness, or the re-attack of damp-heat evils on body with insufficient qi and blood. If the color of fur is in yellow and the texture of the fur is grease. It is named the yellow greasy fur (Fig. 2.2.2.2j).

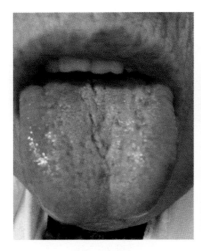 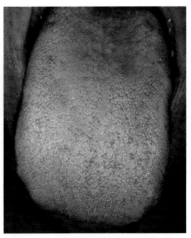

图 2.2.2.2i
Fig. 2.2.2.2i

图 2.2.2.2j
Fig. 2.2.2.2j

苔黄而干燥，甚至苔干而硬，颗粒粗大，扪之糙手者，称黄糙苔（图 2.2.2.2k ）；苔黄而干涩，中有裂纹如花瓣状，称黄瓣苔（图 2.2.2.2l）；黄黑相兼，如烧焦的锅巴，称焦黄苔（图 2.2.2.2m）。以上均主邪热伤津，燥结腑实之证。

The coating, dry and yellow, even dry and stiff, with big particles and sand-palpating sensation, is named yellow rough fur (Fig. 2.2.2.2 k). Dry and yellow fur with petal-like fissures in the middle is named yellow petal fur (Fig. 2.2.2.2l). Yellow-black fur like burnt rice crust is called scorched yellow fur (Fig. 2.2.2.2 m). All these suggest pathogenic heat impairing body fluid and excess syndrome of *fu*-organs with dry feces.

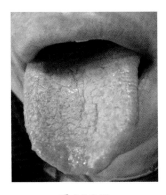 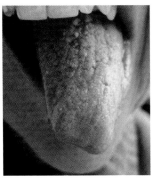 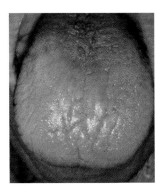

图 2.2.2.2k   图 2.2.2.2l   图 2.2.2.2m
Fig. 2.2.2.2k   Fig. 2.2.2.2l   Fig. 2.2.2.2m

（三）灰黑苔

2.3　Gray-black fur

［舌象特征］苔色呈浅黑，称灰苔（图 2.2.2.3a）；苔色呈深黑，称黑苔（图 2.2.2.3b）。灰苔与黑苔，只是颜色深浅之差别，故并称为灰黑苔。其多由白苔或黄苔转化而来。

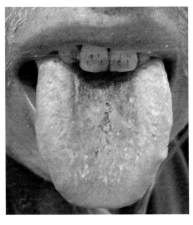 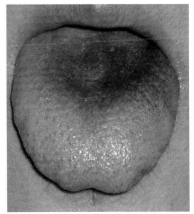

图 2.2.2.3a   图 2.2.2.3b
Fig. 2.2.2.3a   Fig. 2.2.2.3b

［Characteristics of the tongue］The gray fur means that the fur is in the light black color (Fig.2.2.2.3a). The fur being in deep black color is named black fur (Fig.2.2.2.3b). The gray fur and black fur only has difference in light or deep color, always be called as gray-black fur. It is mostly transformed from the white or yellow fur.

［临床意义］主阴寒内盛，或里热炽盛。

［Clinical significance］It is mostly resulted from the excessive internal yin-cold and heat.

［**机理分析**］苔质的润燥是辨别灰黑苔寒热属性的重要指征。在寒湿病中出现灰黑苔，多由白苔转变而成，其舌苔灰黑必湿润多津（图 2.2.2.3c）；在热性病中出现，多由黄苔转变而来，其舌苔灰黑必干燥无津液（图 2.2.2.3d）。

［Mechanism analysis］Moistness and dryness of fur texture is the important index for the clinical doctor to judge the gray-black fur resulting from whether cold or heat. The gray-black fur in disease of cold-dampness is mostly transformed from white fur. It should be moist and there is much fluid on the surface (Fig.2.2.2.3c). The gray-black fur in cases of hot nature is usually transformed from the yellow fur. It should be dry and there is no fluid on the surface (Fig.2.2.2.3d).

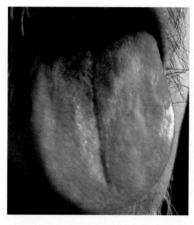 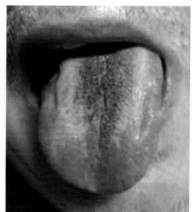

图 2.2.2.3c   图 2.2.2.3d
Fig. 2.2.2.3c   Fig. 2.2.2.3d

第三章 舌诊临床应用

Chapter 3 Clinical Application of the Tongue Diagnosis

　　舌诊是通过观察患者舌质和舌苔的变化，以诊察疾病的方法。《临证验舌法》曰："凡内外杂症，亦无一不呈其形，著其气于舌……据舌以分虚实，而虚实不爽焉；据舌以分阴阳，而阴阳不谬焉；据舌以分脏腑，配主方，则脏腑不差，主方不误焉。危急疑难之顷，往往症无可参，脉无可按，而惟以舌为凭；妇女幼稚之病，往往闻之无息，问之无声，而惟有舌可验。"凡脏腑的虚实、气血的盛衰、津液的盈亏、胃气的存亡、病情的浅深、病邪的性质、预后的吉凶，都能较为客观地从舌象上反映出来。舌象随着病情的变化而变化，舌诊在诊治临床变化多端的疾病中得到广泛应用，发挥着重要作用。

　　Tongue diagnosis is a diagnostic method by which the patient's changes of tongue texture and tongue fur are observed. In the book *Tongue Diagnosis for Clinical Practice*, it stated that "All internal, external, and miscellaneous diseases can be reflected on the tongue without exception... deficiency or excess, yin or yang, sick viscera, and prescriptions can be distinguished exactly according to the tongue manifestations. In some emergencies and difficult cases, it's not unusual that no symptom and pulse can be referred to. Likewise, for women's or children's disease, it's not unusual that listening, smelling, or inquiring method isn't effective. Therefore, only tongue diagnosis can be relied on for the above-mentioned two situations." Tongue manifestation can objectively reflect such aspects as deficiency or excess of the viscera, exuberance or decline of qi-blood, waxing or waning of body fluid, existence or exhaustion of stomach-qi, severity or nature of the disease, favorable or unfavorable prognosis, etc. And the changes of tongue manifestation vary with the development of disease condition. Therefore, tongue diagnosis is widely used and plays an important role in diagnosing and treating various changeable diseases.

第一节　常见证候的舌象特征

Section 1 Tongue Manifestation Characteristics of Common Syndrome

一、气虚证

1. Qi deficiency syndrome

气虚证指元气不足，气的推动、固摄、防御、气化等功能减退，或脏器组织的功能减退，以气短、乏力、神疲、脉虚等为主要表现的虚弱证候。

Qi deficiency syndrome is mainly manifested by shortness of breath, lack of strength, mental fatigue and weak pulse, etc., which is caused by insufficient original qi with hypofunction of qi in promoting, consolidating, defending and transforming, or hypofunction of *zang-fu* organs and tissues.

［主要症状］气短声低，少气懒言，或咳喘无力，神疲乏力，面色淡白，脉虚无力，或头晕目眩，自汗，动则诸症加剧等。

［Main manifestation］Shortness of breath with faint low voice, shortage of qi and disinclination to talk, or faint coughing, mental fatigue and lack of strength, pale complexion, weak pulse or dizziness, spontaneous sweating, all symptoms are deteriorated after movement.

［舌象特征］其舌象异常多表现在舌色上，轻者可无明显异常，稍重者舌色淡白少华，甚者舌象淡白胖嫩。（图3.1.1.1a，图3.1.1.1b）

［Characteristics of the tongue］The abnormality of tongue manifestation

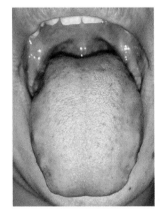
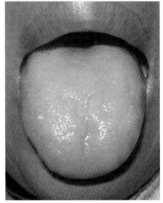

图 3.1.1.1a　　　　　　图 3.1.1.1b
Fig.3.1.1.1a　　　　　　Fig. 3.1.1.1b

is mainly manifested by the tongue color. The tongue color of the mild patients may show no obvious abnormality, the slightly severe ones may look pale and lack of luster, and the severe ones may look pale with enlarged and tender tongue (Fig.3.1.1.1a, Fig.3.1.1.1b).

二、血虚证
2. Blood deficiency syndrome

血虚证指血液亏虚，不能濡养脏腑、经络、组织，以面、睑、唇、舌色白，脉细为主要表现的虚弱证候。

Blood deficiency syndrome is mainly manifested by pale complexion, eyelids, lips, and tongue due to insufficient blood failing to nourish the *zang-fu* organs, meridians and tissues, as well as thready pulse, which is caused by insufficient blood.

［**主要症状**］面色淡白或萎黄，眼睑、口唇、爪甲、舌质的颜色淡白，或头晕眼花，两目干涩，心悸失眠，多梦，健忘，神疲，肢体麻木，或妇女月经量少色淡，延期甚或闭经，脉细无力。

［Main manifestation］Pale or shallow yellow complexion, pale eyelids, lips, nails and tongue, dizziness, dry eyes, palpitation and insomnia, dreaminess, amnesia, mental fatigue, numbness of limbs, scanty menstruation with light color, delayed menorrhea, amenorrhea, and thready and weak pulse.

［**舌象特征**］其舌象异常亦表现在舌色上，轻者舌色淡白无华，甚者白多红少，血色几无（图 3.1.1.2a，图 3.1.1.2b ）。

［Characteristics of the tongue］The abnormality of tongue manifestation is mainly manifested by the tongue color. The tongue color of the mild patients may look pale and lack of luster, the severe ones may look pale and no red at all (Fig.3.1.1.2a, Fig.3.1.1.2b).

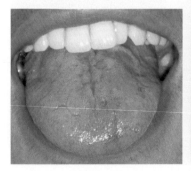 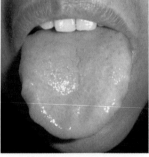

图 3.1.1.2a   图 3.1.1.2b
Fig.3.1.1.2a   Fig. 3.1.1.2b

三、阴虚证

3. Yin deficiency syndrome

阴虚证指体内阴液亏少而无以制阳，滋润、濡养等功能减退，以咽干、五心烦热、脉细数等为主要表现的虚热证候。

Yin deficiency syndrome is mainly manifested by dry throat, vexing heat in chest palms and soles, and thready rapid pulse caused by deficient yin fluid failing to suppress yang with hypofunction of nourishing and moistening.

［主要症状］形体消瘦，口干咽燥，两颧潮红，五心烦热，午后或入夜潮热，甚则热如骨蒸，盗汗，小便短黄，大便干结，脉细数。

［Main manifestation］Emaciation, dry mouth and throat, tidal reddening of the cheeks, vexing heat in chest, palms and soles, afternoon or nighttime tidal fever, steaming bone fever, night sweat, short and dark urine, dry stool, even thready and rapid pulse.

［舌象特征］其典型舌象表现为舌红少苔（图 3.1.1.3a），各类剥苔亦是常见。其中前剥者多为心肺阴虚（图 3.1.1.3b），中剥者多为脾胃阴虚（图 3.1.1.3c），后剥者多为肾阴虚（图 3.1.1.3d）。

［Characteristics of the tongue］The typical manifestation of tongue is red tongue with scanty fur (Fig.3.1.1.3a), and various kinds of peeling fur are also commonly seen. Peeling fur on tip of the tongue indicates yin deficiency of heart-lung (Fig.3.1.1.3b), peeling fur on center of the tongue indicates yin deficiency of spleen-stomach (Fig.3.1.1.3c). While, on root of the tongue indicates kidney yin deficiency (Fig. 3.1.1.3d).

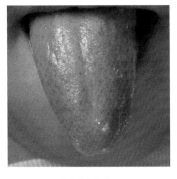 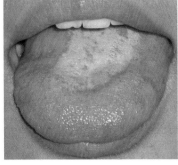

图 3.1.1.3a　　　　　　　　图 3.1.1.3b
Fig.3.1.1.3a　　　　　　　　Fig.3.1.1.3b

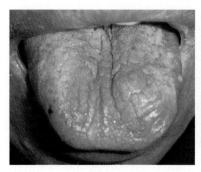 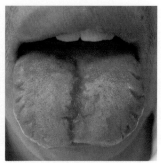

图 3.1.1.3c   图 3.1.1.3d
Fig.3.1.1.3c   Fig.3.1.1.3d

四、阳虚证

4. Yang deficiency syndrome

阳虚证指体内阳气亏损，机体失却温养，推动、蒸腾、气化等作用减退，以畏冷肢凉为主要表现的虚寒证候。

Yang deficiency syndrome is mainly manifested by fear of cold and cold limbs, which is caused by insufficient yang qi failing to warm the body with hypofunction of qi in promoting, transpirating and transforming.

［**主要症状**］畏寒肢凉，口淡不渴，或喜热饮，或自汗，小便清长或尿少不利，大便稀薄，脉沉迟无力，或可见细数无力。可兼见神疲、乏力、气短等气虚表现。

［Main manifestation］Fear of cold, cold extremes, tastelessness in mouth without thirst or prefer hot drinks, spontaneous perspiration, clear abundant urine or scanty urine with difficult urination, loose stool, deep, slow and weak pulse, or thready, rapid and weak pulse. Concurrently, symptoms of qi deficiency can be seen such as mental fatigue, lack of strength, and shortness of breath.

［**舌象特征**］偏虚寒者，舌色淡白而苔白（图 3.1.1.4a）；阳虚而水湿内盛者，舌色淡白胖嫩，苔白而多湿滑（图 3.1.1.4b）；阳虚兼见气血不畅者，舌淡紫而胖（图 3.1.1.4c）。

［Characteristics of the tongue］The tongue of deficiency-cold type may look pale, with white fur (Fig.3.1.1.4a). Yang deficiency with fluid retention type may look pale with enlarged shape and tender texture, white, moisten and slippery fur (Fig.3.1.1.4b). Yang deficiency with qi-blood stagnation type may look pale purple with enlarged shape (Fig.3.1.1.4c).

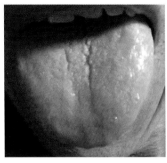

图 3.1.1.4a
Fig.3.1.1.4a

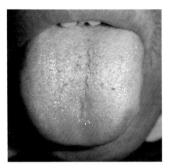

图 3.1.1.4b
Fig.3.1.1.4b

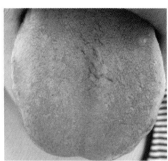

图 3.1.1.4c
Fig.3.1.1.4c

五、津液亏虚证

5. Fluid and humor deficiency syndrome

津液亏虚证指体内津液亏少，脏腑、组织、官窍失却濡润、滋养、充盈，以口渴尿少、口、鼻、唇、舌、皮肤、大便干燥为主要表现的证候。

Fluid and humor deficiency syndrome is mainly manifested by thirst with oliguria, dry mouth, nose, lips, tongue and skin as well as dry stool which is caused by insufficient body fluid failing to moisten, nourish, and saturate the *zang-fu* organs, tissues, and orifices.

［主要症状］口、鼻、唇、舌、咽喉、皮肤等干燥，甚则皮肤枯瘪而乏弹性，眼球下陷，口渴欲饮，小便短少而黄，大便干燥，脉细或细数无力等。

［Main manifestation］Dry mouth, nose, lips, tongue and dry skin, etc., even withered and inelastic skin, sunken eyes, thirst with desire to drink, scatty yellow urine, dry stool, thready, rapid and weak pulse.

［舌象特征］一般以舌上干燥少津为主要变现（图 3.1.1.5a），其重者可见舌质红而苔干燥（图 3.1.1.5b）。

［Characteristics of the tongue］The tongue manifestation of this syndrome is mainly manifested by dry tongue with little fluid (Fig.3.1.1.5a). The severe one may

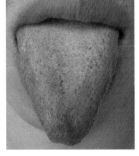

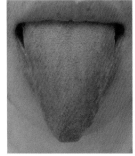

图 3.1.1.5a
Fig.3.1.1.5a

图 3.1.1.5b
Fig. 3.1.1.5b

show red tongue with dry fur (Fig.3.1.1.5b).

六、气滞证

6. Qi stagnation syndrome

气滞证指人体某一部分或某一脏腑、经络的气机阻滞，运行不畅，以胀闷疼痛为主要表现的证候。

Qi stagnation syndrome is mainly manifested by distention pain due to qi stagnation and its unsmooth movement in *zang-fu* organs or meridians.

［**主要症状**］胸胁、脘腹等处或损伤部位的胀闷或疼痛，疼痛性质可为胀痛、窜痛、攻痛，程度时轻时重，部位不定，按之一般无形，疼痛常随嗳气、肠鸣、矢气等而减轻，或随情绪变化而增减，脉多弦。

［Main manifestation］Fullness or distention pain in chest, hypochondrium, stomach and abdomen or injured parts. The characteristic of the pain may be distending, scurrying or attacking, with different degree and location. The pain feels intangible when touches it, and may relieve after belching, borborygmus and flatus. It also varies with emotion changes, and mostly with wiry pulse.

［**舌象特征**］舌象可无明显变化；脘腹胀闷则多见舌淡红，苔白微厚腻或苔白腻而偏燥（图 3.1.1.6a）；若气滞兼血行不畅者，亦可见舌质淡紫或兼有瘀点（图 3.1.1.6b）。

［Characteristics of the tongue］The tongue manifestation of this syndrome may show no marked variation. The patients with the symptoms of gastric or abdominal fullness and distention may show light red tongue (Fig.3.1.1.6a), with white, slightly thick and greasy fur, or with white, greasy and slightly dry fur. The patient with qi stagnation and blood unsmoothness may show pale purple tongue or with ecchymosis (Fig.3.1.1.6b).

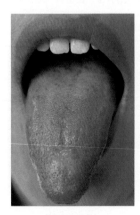

图 3.1.1.6a
Fig.3.1.1.6a

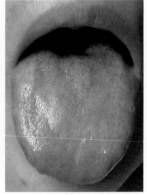

图 3.1.1.6b
Fig.3.1.1.6b

七、血瘀证

7. Blood stasis syndrome

血瘀证指瘀血内阻，血行不畅，以固定刺痛、肿块、出血、瘀血舌脉征为主要表现的证候。

Blood stasis syndrome is mainly manifested by fixed stabbing pain, lump, bleeding, and stasis-signifying tongue and pulse, which is caused by internal accumulation of blood stasis and its unsmooth movement.

［**主要症状**］疼痛，其特点为刺痛、痛处拒按、固定不移，夜间痛甚；肿块，在体表者包块色青紫，腹内者触及质硬而推之不移；出血，色紫暗或夹血块，面色黧黑，肌肤甲错，脉多细涩或结、代。

［Main manifestation］Pain (fixed unpalpable stabbing pain that aggravates at night); lump (cyanotic lump underneath the body surface, or hard fixed abdominal lump); bleeding (of dark purple color or with blood clot, blackish complexion, scaly skin, thready unsmooth pulse, or irregularly or regularly intermittent pulse).

［**舌象特征**］其舌质多淡紫、青紫或紫暗（图 3.1.1.7a），或见舌边瘀斑、舌边舌尖瘀点（图 3.1.1.7b）。其舌下脉络多见青紫、曲张，甚至紫黑（图 3.1.1.7c）。

［Characteristics of the tongue］The tongue may look pale purple, cyanotic or dark purple (Fig.3.1.1.7a), with petechia on the tip and margin of the tongue (Fig.3.1.1.7b). It may show cyanotic, varicose or even dark purple sublingual venation (Fig.3.1.1.7c).

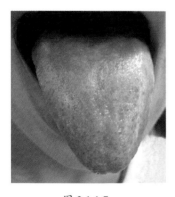 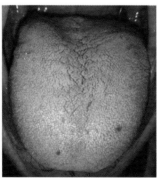 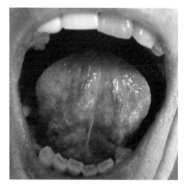

| 图 3.1.1.7a | 图 3.1.1.7a | 图 3.1.1.7a |
| Fig.3.1.1.7a | Fig.3.1.1.7a | Fig.3.1.1.7a |

八、实热证

8. Excess heat syndrome

实热证指邪热亢盛，内外俱实的病证，即感受阳热之邪所致的证候，多因热邪入侵，里热炽盛，或痰瘀、宿食阻滞所致。

Excess heat syndrome refers to the symptoms with the nature of exuberant pathogenic heat and excess in interior and exterior, which is caused by yang-heat invading the body, interior heat exuberance, phlegm-stasis, or food accumulation.

［**主要症状**］发热恶热，喜冷，或局部灼痛，面目红赤，口渴喜冷饮，痰涕黄浊，小便短黄，大便干结，或烦躁不安，甚则神昏谵语，或吐血、衄血，脉数。

［Main manifestation］Fever, aversion to heat and preference for cold, localized burning pain, flushed face and red eyes, thirst with desire to cold drink, yellow turbid phlegm and snivel, scanty yellow urine, dry stool, or restlessness, even unconsciousness and delirious speech, or hematemesis, epistaxis, and rapid pulse.

［**舌象特征**］表热证多见舌淡红苔薄黄（图 3.1.1.8a）；里实热证多见舌红 , 邪热郁久则见舌红苔黄（图 3.1.1.8b）；热盛则舌红苔黄燥（图 3.1.1.8c）；兼有湿邪则多黄腻苔（图 3.1.1.8d）。不同脏腑有热舌象也不同，心肺热证多见舌尖红（图 3.1.1.8e），心火亢盛可见舌尖红碎或生疮疡（图 3.1.1.8f），肝胆热盛则多见舌边红（图 3.1.1.8g）。

［Characteristics of the tongue］The exterior-heat syndrome may show light red tongue with thin yellow fur (Fig.3.1.1.8a). The interior-heat one may show red tongue. Prolonged heat stagnation type may show red tongue with yellow fur (Fig.3.1.1.8b). Exuberant heat may show red tongue with dry yellow fur (Fig.3.1.1.8c), if accompanied with dampness, it may often show yellow greasy fur (Fig.3.1.1.8d). Heat in different *zang-fu* organs also manifests differently. Heart-lung heat syndrome may show red tongue tip (Fig.3.1.1.8e). Exuberance of heart fire type may show red tongue or with sore (Fig.3.1.1.8f). Heat exuberance of liver and gallbladder syndrome may show red margins of the tongue (Fig.3.1.1.8g).

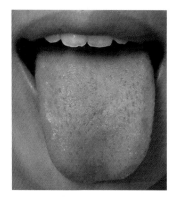

图 3.1.1.8a
Fig.3.1.1.8a

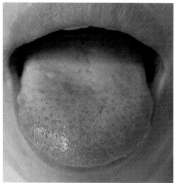

图 3.1.1.8b
Fig.3.1.1.8b

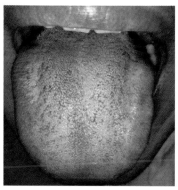

图 3.1.1.8c
Fig.3.1.1.8c

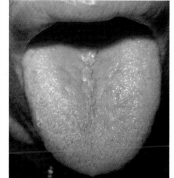

图 3.1.1.8d
Fig.3.1.1.8d

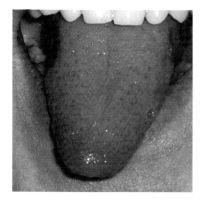

图 3.1.1.8e
Fig.3.1.1.8e

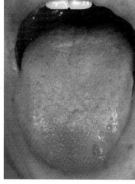

图 3.1.1.8f
Fig.3.1.1.8f

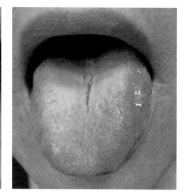

图 3.1.1.8g
Fig.3.1.1.8g

九、实寒证

9. Excess cold syndrome

实寒证指因外界寒邪侵袭，或过服生冷寒凉所致，以起病急骤，体质壮实，符合寒证、实证特点为主要表现的证候。

Excess cold syndrome refers to excess syndrome and cold syndrome with rapid onset and robust constitution, which is caused by pathogenic cold attacking the body, or over-intake of raw and cold food.

［**主要症状**］畏寒恶寒，喜暖，或局部冷痛；面色淡白或青，四肢不温，口淡不渴；痰、涎、涕清稀；或小便清长，大便稀溏，脉迟或紧。

［Main manifestation］Fear of cold, aversion to cold, preference for warmth, or localized cold pain; pale or caynotic complexion, cold limbs, tastelessness in the mouth without thirst; clear thin phlegm, saliva, and snivel; clear abundant urine, loose stool, slow or tight pulse.

［**舌象特征**］表寒证见舌淡红，苔薄白或白而稍厚（图 3.1.1.9a）；里寒证见舌色淡白，苔白而滑润（图 3.1.1.9b）；寒邪郁久则多见苔白腻而湿滑（图 3.1.1.9c）。

［Characteristics of the tongue］Exterior-cold syndrome may show light red tongue, with thin white fur, or slightly thick white fur (Fig3.1.1.9a). Interior-cold syndrome may manifest as pale tongue with white, slippery and moist fur (Fig3.1.1.9b). Prolonged stagnated cold type may show white, greasy, wet and slippery fur (Fig3.1.1.9c).

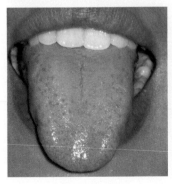 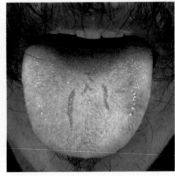 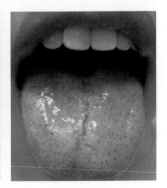

图 3.1.1.9a   图 3.1.1.9b   图 3.1.1.9c
Fig.3.1.1.9a   Fig.3.1.1.9b   Fig.3.1.1.9c

十、痰湿证

10. Phlegm-dampness syndrome

痰湿证指因脾虚失运，津液输布失常，水湿内停所致湿浊内停，日久成痰，导致痰浊内阻或流窜，以咳吐痰多、胸闷、呕恶、眩晕、体胖，或局部有圆滑包块，苔腻、脉滑为主要表现的证候。

Phlegm-dampness syndrome is mainly manifested by coughing with profuse phlegm, chest congestion, nausea and vomit, dizziness, obesity, or localized smooth lumps, greasy fur, and slippery pulse. It is caused by dysfunction of spleen in transportation and transformation, abnormal distribution of body fluid, and internal retention of water and dampness, which further induces internal obstruction or scurry of phlegm turbidity or dampness turbidity.

［**主要症状**］其表现多端，可见于全身多个脏腑和部位。痰湿停于肺，则见咳嗽喘息、胸闷咳痰；停于胃，则见食少纳呆，胃脘闷痞，甚恶呕痰涎；停于肌肤或身体局部位置，出现圆滑柔韧的包块；还可痰蒙心神导致神昏，或神志错乱而为癫、狂、痴、痫；或头晕目眩；或形体肥胖；脉多濡滑。

［Main manifestation］The manifestation is various according to different organs and positions. If phlegm-dampness retains in the lung, cough, dyspnea, chest congestion and expectoration of phlegm will appear; if in the stomach, there will be such symptoms as reduced appetite, anorexia, gastric distention,or even vomiting of phlegm or saliva; if under the skin or localized part of the body,smooth round lumps occur. The severe ones may show unconsciousness due to phlegm clouding heart spirit, even mental abnormality such as pyschosis, mania, dementia, epilepsy, dizziness, obesity, and soggy slippery pulse.

［**舌象特征**］该证最主要的特征是腻苔。湿浊或痰浊内盛者苔黏腻或垢腻（图3.1.1.10a）；其痰湿热化多见舌苔黄腻（图3.1.1.10b），热重多见舌红苔黄腻而干燥（图3.1.1.10c），湿重则苔黄腻而湿滑（图3.1.1.10d）；其痰湿寒化主要表现为舌苔白腻，寒盛则舌色淡白苔白厚腻而润（图3.1.1.10e），湿盛则苔白腻而多湿滑（图3.1.1.10f），兼有阳虚水泛者则多见舌质色淡而胖嫩，苔白腻而多水湿（图3.1.1.10g）。

［Characteristics of the tongue］The main characteristic of this syndrome is greasy fur. Internal exuberance of phlegm turbidity or dampness turbidity may show sticky greasy fur or dirty fur (Fig.3.1.1.10a); heat transformation of phlegm-dampness may show yellow greasy fur (Fig.3.1.1.10b), of which, preponderance of heat may show red tongue with yellow, greasy and dry fur (Fig.3.1.1.10c), whereas preponderance of dampness may manifest yellow, greasy, wet and slippery fur (Fig.3.1.1.10d); cold transformation of phlegm-dampness may show white greasy fur, of which, cold preponderance may manifest pale tongue with white, thick, greasy and moist fur (Fig.3.1.1.10e), whereas dampness preponderance may manifest white, greasy, wet and slippery fur (Fig.3.1.1.10f), if it is accompanied with yang deficiency and water diffusion, there may show pale, enlarged, tender and watery tongue with white greasy fur (Fig.3.1.1.10g).

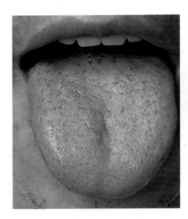
图 3.1.1.10a
Fig.3.1.1.10a

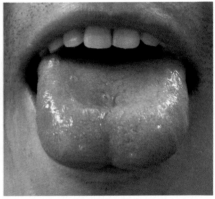
图 3.1.1.10b
Fig.3.1.1.10b

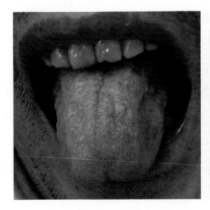
图 3.1.1.10c
Fig.3.1.1.10c

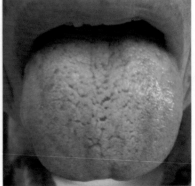
图 3.1.1.10d
Fig.3.1.1.10d

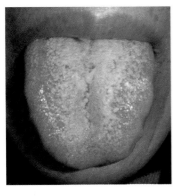
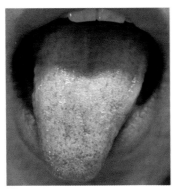
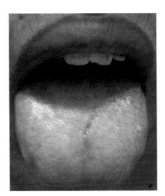

图 3.1.1.10e
Fig.3.1.1.10e

图 3.1.1.10f
Fig.3.1.1.10f

图 3.1.1.10g
Fig.3.1.1.10g

十一、食积证

11. Food accumulation syndrome

食积证是指饮食不节，伤及胃肠或脾虚失运致饮食停滞胃肠所表现的证候。

Food accumulation refers to the symptom of food retention in stomach and intestines, which is caused by improper diet damaging stomach and intestines, or spleen deficiency failing to transport and transform water and food nutrients.

［**主要症状**］脘腹饱胀或脐腹疼痛拒按，吞酸嗳腐，恶闻食臭；或恶心呕吐，或便秘，或腹痛腹泻；舌苔厚浊，脉滑。

［Main manifestation］Epigastric fullness or distention, or unpalpable umbilical and abdominal pain, acid regurgitation, belching with fetid odour; or nausea and vomiting, or constipation, or abdominal pain and diarrhea; thick and turbid fur, and slippery pulse.

［**舌象特征**］暴饮暴食，壅塞胃肠所致者，多舌红苔厚腐浊（图 3.1.1.11a）；脾虚失运，积食久停所致者，多舌淡苔腐或滑腻（图 3.1.1.11b）。

［Characteristics of the tongue］The crapulence cases with food congestion in stomach and intestines may show red tongue with thick, putrid and turbid fur (Fig.3.1.1.11a); the cases with prolonged food accumulation due to spleen deficiency may show pale tongue with putrid or slippery greasy fur (Fig.3.1.1.11b).

79

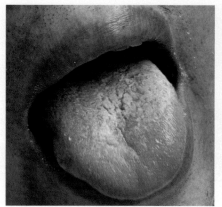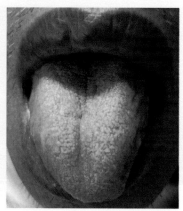

图 3.1.1.11a　　　　　　　　　　图 3.1.1.11b
Fig.3.1.1.11a　　　　　　　　　　Fig.3.1.1.11b

第二节　临床病证举隅

Section 2　Examples of Clinical Medical Records

一、心系病证

1. Heart System Syndrome

（一）心悸 – 心阳不足证

1.1　Palpitation: syndrome of heart yang deficiency

患者李某，男，35 岁，心中悸动 1 年加重 10 天，于 2008 年 4 月 7 日就诊。

Patient Li, male, 35 years old, had been suffering from palpitation for one year and the symptom aggravated 10 days ago. Then he visited a doctor on April 7, 2008.

患者于 1 年前因突发心悸不安，于当地医院查心电图示"频发室性早搏"，予口服倍他乐克、肌苷等药物治疗，症状有所减轻。10 天前患者因过度劳累而心悸不安症状加重，遂来就诊。刻诊：神疲乏力，面色萎黄，心悸频发，胸中发空，气短不得接续，动则汗出，畏寒怕冷，寐差易醒，纳食可，小便平，大便偏溏，舌质淡紫，苔水滑（图 3.2.1.1a），脉弦细而有结象。

The patient suffered from sudden palpitation one year ago and ECG of the local hospital showed frequent ventricular premature beat (FVPB) in local hospital. He was given betaloc and inosine, etc. for treatment and the palpitation was alleviated. The symptom was aggravated 10 days ago because of overstrain, and then the patient came to seek treatment. Present symptoms: fatigue, shallow yellow complexion, frequent palpitation, emptiness in heart, shortness of breath and dyspnea, sweating with movement, aversion to cold, poor sleep and easy wake-up, normal diet and urine, loose stool, pale purple tongue with slippery fur, (Fig.3.2.1.1a), wiry thread and irregularly intermittent pulse.

西医诊断：室心早搏。

Western medicine diagnosis: frequent ventricular premature beat (FVPB).

中医诊断：心悸。

TCM diagnosis: palpitation.

辨证：胸阳不振，气机痹阻证。

Syndrome differentiation: chest yang weakness and qi movement obstruction.

治疗：通阳化饮，裨益心气。

Treatment: activating yang and resolving fluid retention, replenishing heart qi.

处方：苓桂术甘汤加减：党参 15g，茯苓 20g，桂枝 10g，白术 15g，炙甘草 8g，丹参 15g，沙参 10g，麦冬 10g。7 剂，日 1 剂，水煎，分 2 次温服。

Prescription: modified *Linggui Zhugan* Decoction.

Dangshen 15g, fuling 20g, guizhi 10g, baizhu 15g, zhigancao 8g, danshen 15g, shashen 10g, maidong 10g.

Seven doses and one dose a day, decoction, take twice warmly.

证候分析：胸阳不振，气机痹阻，心脉不畅，则心悸、失眠；阳虚温煦、摄纳失职，动则汗出；阳虚不运，水湿不化，停滞四肢，则神疲乏力；阳虚温煦失职，则畏寒；面色萎黄，舌质淡紫，苔水滑，脉弦细而有结象，乃胸阳不振，水饮内停之象。

Syndrome analysis: chest yang weakness, qi movement obstruction and unsmooth heart vessels result in palpitation and insomnia. Yang deficiency leads to body's abnormal warming and consolidating functions, therefore, symptoms such as sweating with movement and aversion to cold appear. Yang deficiency fails to transform the water, so water retains in the limbs and causes fatigue. Symptoms such as shallow yellow complexion, pale purple tongue with slippery fur, wiry thready and irregularly intermittent pulse are manifestations of chest yang weakness and water retention.

2008 年 4 月 14 日二诊：心悸明显减轻，胸中已不觉发空，舌淡，苔白滑（图 3.2.1.1b），脉细。守前方继服 10 剂而愈。

Second visit on April 14, 2008: the palpitation was obviously relieved, and he felt no emptiness in the heart. The tongue was pale with white slippery fur (Fig. 3.2.1.1b), and the pulse was thready. The patient was asked to take the previous prescription for 10 doses and he was in recovery.

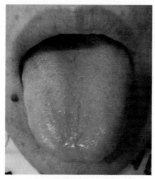

图 3.2.1.1a   图 3.2.1.1b
Fig.3.2.1.1a   Fig.3.2.1.1b

（二）心悸 – 心阳虚衰证

1.2 Palpitation: syndrome of heart yang debilitation

患者刘某，女，59 岁，咳喘、心悸 3 月加重 1 周，于 2014 年 12 月 11 日就诊。

Patient Liu, female, 59 years old, had been suffering from cough, asthma and palpitation for 3 months and the symptoms aggravated one week ago. Then she visited a doctor on December 11, 2014.

患者 3 个月前因咳喘、心悸于某医院就诊，诊断为肺源性心脏病，住院治疗好转而出院。7 天前患者因劳累、受寒而发心悸、咳喘，遂来就诊。刻诊：面色晦暗，精神欠佳，咳嗽、喘息，胸闷、心悸，夜间不能平卧，心下坚满，双下肢浮肿，纳差，夜寐不安，小便量少，大便稀溏，舌质暗紫，苔薄白（图 3.2.1.2a），脉沉细。

The patient was treated in a hospital for cough, asthma and palpitation 3 months ago. She was diagnosed as pulmonary heart disease, then hospitalized and discharged from the hospital when getting better. Seven days ago, the patient came for treatment because of cough, asthma and palpitation induced by fatigue and cold attack. Present symptoms: dull complexion, poor spirit, coughing, asthma, chest distress, palpitation, difficult lying flat at night, fullness and hardness below the heart, lower limbs edema, poor diet, restless sleep, scanty urine, loose stool, dark purple tongue with thin and white fur (Fig.3.2.1.2a), and deep thready pulse.

西医诊断：肺源性心脏病。

Western medicine diagnosis: pulmonary heart disease.

中医诊断：心悸。

TCM diagnosis: palpitation.

辨证：心阳不振，水气凌心证。

Syndrome differentiation: weakness of heart yang and water pathogen attacking heart.

治疗：温阳化气，止咳平喘。

Treatment: warming yang and transforming qi, relieving cough and dyspnea.

处方：桂枝芍药知母汤合麻黄附子细辛汤加减：桂枝 10g，麻黄 6g，附子 8g（先煎），细辛 3g，茯苓 15g，大腹皮 15g，夜交藤 30g，柏子仁 15g，麦芽 15g，紫菀 10g，黄芪 15g，防己 10g，泽泻 10g，炙甘草 5g。7 剂，日 1 剂，水煎，分 2 次温服。

Prescription: modified *Guizhi Shaoyao Zhimu* Decoction together with *Mahuang Fuzi Xixin* Decoction.

Guizhi 10g, mahuang 6g, fuzi 8g (decocted first), xixin 3g, fuling 15g, dafupi 15g, yejiaoteng 30g, baiziren 15g, maiya 15g, ziwan 10g, huangqi 15g, fangji 10g, zexie 10g, zhigancao 5g.

Seven doses and one dose a day, decoction, take twice warmly.

证候分析：心阳不振，水饮凌心，扰乱心神，则心悸、失眠；水饮不循常道，阻滞气机，则胸闷、心下坚满；胸胁阻滞较甚，则夜间不能平卧；水饮上犯肺系，肺失宣降，则咳嗽、喘息；阳气虚衰，不能温化水湿，膀胱气化失司，故小便短少、大便溏泻；饮溢四肢，饮为阴邪，故下肢浮肿；阳虚不化，失却温煦，则舌质暗紫；苔薄白，脉沉细，为水饮内停之象。

Syndrome analysis: weakness of heart yang together with water pathogen attacking heart and disturbing mind lead to palpitation and insomnia. The abnormal flow of water and fluid-retention blocks qi movement, so chest distress, and fullness and hardness below the heart appeared. Serious blockage in the chest and hypochondrium makes difficult lying flat at night. Water pathogen upward invading lung induces the lung's dysfunction in dispersing and descending, then cough and asthma occur. Yang deficiency fails to transform the water, which causes the failure of the bladder's qi transformation, therefore, scanty urine and loose stool occur. On the other hand, the overflow of fluid-retention to four limbs and its yin nature triggers low limb edema. Yang deficiency leading to body's abnormal warming function explains dark purple tongue. Thin and white tongue fur along with deep thready pulse manifests fluid-retention stagnating in the interior.

2014 年 12 月 18 日二诊：患者精神转佳，心下坚满变软，喘息已平，心悸症状减轻，下肢浮肿稍减，舌淡紫，苔白（图 3.2.1.2b），脉沉。继以温阳益气、调补心肾方药善后。

Second visit on December 18, 2014: the patient's spirit had been lifted, fullness and hardness below the heart softened, asthma disappeared, and palpitation and lower limb edema relieved. The tongue was pale purple with white fur (Fig.3.2.1.2b) and the pulse deep. The prescription of warming yang and replenishing qi as well as regulating the heart and the kidney was administered for rehabilitation.

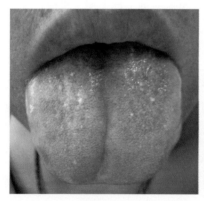 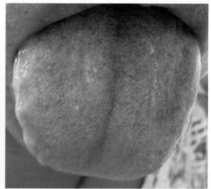

图 3.2.1.2a 　　　　　　　　　　　　图 3.2.1.2b
Fig.3.2.1.2a 　　　　　　　　　　　　Fig.3.2.1.2b

（三）心悸 – 心阴亏虚证

1.3　Palpitation: syndrome of heart yin deficiency

患者黄某，男，47 岁，心悸怔忡 2 年加重半月，于 2013 年 6 月 3 日就诊。

Patient Huang, male, 47 years old, had been suffering from palpitation and severe palpitation for 2 years and the symptoms aggravated half a month ago. Then he visited a doctor on June 3, 2013.

患者 2 年前因冒雨后感冒发热，遂出现心慌不已，当地医院诊为"病毒性心肌炎"，间断服稳心颗粒治疗。近半月来，患者自感心慌不宁，寐差，遂来就诊。刻诊：精神不振，自我感觉心慌不宁，语声无力，纳可，夜寐多梦，阵发性汗出，小便平，大便干，2 日一行，舌红绛，少苔（图 3.2.1.3a），脉结代。心电图示：窦性心律伴房性早搏。

The patient had been in a state of flusteredness because of a cold and fever after he caught the rain 2 years ago. He was diagnosed as viral myocarditis in the local hospital and treated with *Wenxin* Granule intermittently. In recent half a month, the patient felt flusteredness, anxious and insomnia, so he came for treatment. Present symptoms: dispiritedness, flusteredness and anxiety, weak voice, normal diet, dreaminess, paroxysmal perspiration, normal urine, dry stool with defecation every 2 days, red crimson tongue with little fur (Fig.3.2.1.3a), and irregular intermittent or intermittent pulse. Electrocardiogram (ECG): sinus heart rhythm with atrial premature beat.

西医诊断：心肌炎。

Western medicine diagnosis: myocarditis.

中医诊断：心悸。

TCM diagnosis: palpitation.

辨证：心阴亏虚，心脉失养证。

Syndrome differentiation: heart yin deficiency and heart vessels malnutrition.

治疗：益气养阴，化瘀宁神。

Treatment: replenishing qi and nourishing yin, removing blood stasis and tranquilizing mind.

处方：天王补心丹加减：黄芪 20g，丹参 30g，北沙参 20g，太子参 10g，麦冬 15g，五味子 10g，茯神 10g，柏子仁 15g，煅龙骨 30g（先煎），煅牡蛎 30g（先煎），琥珀末 3g（冲服）。7 剂，日 1 剂，水煎，分 2 次温服。

Prescription: modified *Tianwang Buxin* Powder.

Huangqi 20g, danshen 30g, beishashen 20g, taizishen 10g, maidong 15g, wuweizi 10g, fushen 10g, baiziren 15g, duanlonggu 30g (decocted first), duanmuli 30g (decocted first), hupomo 3g (take medicine with water).

Seven doses and one dose a day, decoction, take twice warmly.

证候分析：心阴亏虚，不能制阳，心阳偏亢，扰乱心神，则心悸怔忡、失眠；心阳迫津外泄，则汗出；阴液不足，则便干；舌红、少苔，脉结代，为心阴不足之明证。

Syndrome analysis: heart yin deficiency fails to restrict heart yang, and heart yang hyperactivity disturbs mind, therefore, palpitation, severe palpitation and insomnia appear. Heart yang forces the fluid outward, so there is paroxysmal perspiration. Insufficient fluid causes dry stool. Red crimson tongue with little fur, and irregular intermittent or regular intermittent pulse are manifestations of heart yin deficiency.

2013 年 6 月 10 日二诊：精神好转，心慌症状减轻，面色转润，夜寐梦减，偶有头晕，纳差，舌红，少苔（图 3.2.1.3b），脉细而结代。原方加升麻 10g、法半夏 10g、陈皮 6g，继服 7 剂。

Second visit on June 10, 2013: dispiritedness, flusteredness and dreaminess were relieved, and the complexion turned lustrous. Other symptoms included occasional dizziness, poor diet, red tongue with little fur (Fig.3.2.1.3b), thready, irregular intermittent or regular intermittent pulse. The previous prescription is used for treatment with the addition of shengma 10g, fabanxia 10g, and chenpi 6g, 7 doses.

2013 年 6 月 17 日三诊：以上诸症均好转，以柏子养心汤善后。

Third visit on June 17, 2013: all of the above symptoms were improved, and *Baizi Yangxin* Decoction was prescribed to consolidate the effect.

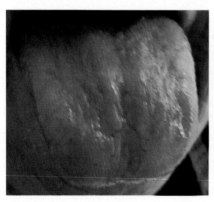 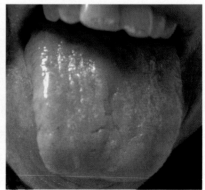

图 3.2.1.3a   图 3.2.1.3b
Fig.3.2.1.3a   Fig.3.2.1.3b

（四）心悸 – 气虚血瘀证

1.4 Palpitation: syndrome of qi deficiency and blood stasis

患者万某，男，67 岁，反复胸闷心慌 5 年余加重 1 天，于 2017 年 4 月 21 日就诊。

Patient Wan, male, 67 years old, had been suffering from repeated chest distress and flusteredness for more than 5 years and the symptoms aggravated one day ago, and he came to visit the doctor on April 21, 2017.

患者既往有高血压病史，最高达 180/90mmHg，5 年前反复出现胸闷心慌症状，未系统治疗。1 天前患者胸闷、心慌症状加重，遂来就诊。刻诊：胸闷心慌，稍动则心慌不已，稍感头痛头晕，左侧颈部疼痛，无咳嗽、咯痰，无恶心、呕吐，右脚趾麻木，易汗出，纳食可，夜寐安，大小便正常，舌质暗红，苔薄黄根部腻（图 3.2.1.4a），脉细涩。常规心电图示：窦性心律；完全性右束支传导阻滞。心脏彩超示：左房增大，左室舒张功能减退。头颅磁共振示：多发脑白质缺血性改变。

The patient had a history of hypertension, with a maximum of 180/90mmHg. He had recurrent chest distress and flusteredness 5 years ago without systematic treatment. He came to visit the doctor because of chest distress and flusteredness aggravated one day ago. Present symptoms: chest distress, flusteredness that aggravates with movement, headache and dizziness, pain in the left neck, no cough and expectoration, no nausea and vomiting, numbness of the right toes, easy sweating, normal appetite, normal sleep, normal urine and stool, dark red tongue, thin yellow fur with greasy in the tongue root (Fig.3.2.1.4a), thin and unsmooth pulse. Routine electrocardiogram showed: sinus rhythm; complete right bundle branch block. UCG showed: left atrial enlargement, hypofunction of diastolic function of the left ventricular. Cranial magnetic resonance showed: ischemic changes of multiple cerebral white matter.

西医诊断：心律失常。

Western medicine diagnosis: arrhythmia.

中医诊断：心悸。

TCM diagnosis: palpitation.

辨证：气虚血瘀，心脉不畅证。

Syndrome differentiation: qi deficiency and blood stasis, heart vessel obstruction.

治疗：益气养心，活血化瘀。

Treatment: replenishing qi and nourishing heart, activating blood and resolving stasis.

处方：血府逐瘀汤加减：红参 10g，黄芪 15g，当归 10g，生地黄 12g，桃仁 10g，红花 10g，赤芍 10g，牡丹皮 10g，鸡血藤 15g，三七 10g，枳壳 10g，炒白术 15g，茯苓 10g。7 剂，日 1 剂，水煎，分 2 次温服。

Prescription: modified *Xuefu Zhuyu* Decoction.

Hongshen 10g, huangqi 10g, danggui 10g, shengdihuang 10g, taoren 10g, honghua 10g, chishao 10g, mudanpi 10g, jixueteng 10g, sanqi 10g, zhiqiao 10g, chaobaizhu 15g, fuling 10g.

Seven doses and one dose a day, decoction, take twice warmly.

证候分析：气虚则血液运行不畅而引起血瘀，瘀血阻滞，新血不生，心失养，则心神不宁、心慌、心悸；气虚固摄失职，则易汗出；动则耗气，心血不足益甚，则心慌不已；舌质暗红，为瘀血内阻之象；苔黄，乃瘀血阻滞而有化火之势；根部腻，为气虚血瘀，水湿不化而致；脉细涩，乃因气虚无力鼓动脉管，血瘀血流不畅，脉道失充而致。

Syndrome analysis: qi deficiency and unsmooth movement of the blood cause blood stasis, which hinders the generation of the new blood and causes insufficient nourishment of heart spirit, therefore, distraction, flusteredness and palpitation appear. Qi deficiency and abnormal consolidating function of qi causes easy sweating. Movement consumes qi that makes heart blood less sufficient, so flusteredness aggravates with movement. Dark red tongue hints the internal obstruction of blood stasis, while yellow fur shows the obstruction of blood stasis transforming into fire. Greasy fur in the tongue root is caused by qi deficiency and blood stasis as well as the non-transformation of water-dampness. Thin and unsmooth pulse is due to qi deficiency, which fails to propel the blood, causes unsmooth blood circulation and malnutrition of the vessel.

2017 年 4 月 28 日二诊：精神转佳，胸闷症状减轻，无头晕头痛，舌质淡红，苔薄黄（图 3.2.1.4b），脉细。维持原方 7 剂，继续治疗。

Second visit on April 28, 2017: the spirit was improved and chest distress was relieved. There was no dizziness and headache. The tongue was light red with thin yellow fur (Fig.3.2.1.4b), and the pulse was thin. Seven doses of the previous prescription were given for further treatment.

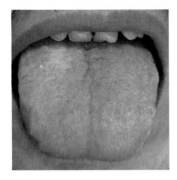 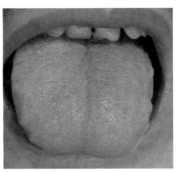

图 3.2.1.4a　　　　　　　　图 3.2.1.4b

Fig.3.2.1.4a　　　　　　　　Fig.3.2.1.4b

（五）心悸 – 心胆气虚证

1.5　Palpitation: syndrome of qi deficiency of heart and gallbladder

患者周某，男，71 岁，心悸不宁 5 年加重 2 个月，于 2015 年 11 月 12 日就诊。

Patient Zhou, male, 71 years old, had been suffering from palpitation and restlessness for 5 years and the symptoms aggravated 2 months ago. Then he came to see the doctor on November 12, 2015.

患者 5 年前因先天性二尖瓣关闭不全手术后出现心悸症状，曾服用多种药物治疗，但症状时好时坏。近 2 个月来，患者因劳累而致心悸不宁症状加重，遂来就诊。刻诊：形体消瘦，焦虑面容，胆小害怕，对巨响敏感，坐卧不安，多梦而易于惊醒，食少纳呆，口淡不渴，二便正常，舌淡，苔黄滑腻（图 3.2.1.5a），脉细略数。

The patient had palpitation after surgery of congenital mitral insufficiency 5 years ago. He took much medicine for treatment, while the symptom of palpitations fluctuated. In recent 2 months, the palpitations and restlessness aggravated with fatigue, so he came for treatment. Present symptoms: emaciation, anxious complexion, timidness, sensitivity to loud noise, restlessness, dreaminess and easy wake-up, poor appetite, tastelessness without thirsty, normal urine and stool, pale tongue with yellow slippery and greasy fur (Fig.3.2.1.5a), thready and slightly rapid pulse.

西医诊断：先天性二尖瓣关闭不全。

Western medicine diagnosis: congenital mitral insufficiency.

中医诊断：心悸。

TCM diagnosis: palpitation.

辨证：心胆气虚，心神不宁证。

Syndrome differentiation: qi deficiency of heart and gallbladder, heart spirit restlessness.

治疗：镇惊定志，养心安神。

Treatment: calming fright and stabilizing mind, nourishing heart and tranquilizing mind.

处方：安神定志丸加减：党参 15g，白术 15g，茯苓 15g，茯神 20g，石菖蒲 10g，远志 10g，龙齿 30g（先煎），夜交藤 30g，陈皮 10g，麦芽 15g，炙甘草 5g。7 剂，日 1 剂，水煎，分 2 次温服。

Prescription: modified *Anshen Dingzhi* Pill.

Dangshen 15g, baizhu 15g, fuling 15g, fushen 20g, shichangpu 10g, yuanzhi 10g, longchi 30g (decocted first), yejiaoteng 30g, chenpi 10g, maiya 15g, zhigancao 5g.

Seven doses and one dose a day, decoction, take twice warmly.

证候分析：心为神舍，心气不足，鼓动无力，心神失养，故心悸不宁，不寐多梦而易惊醒；胆气怯弱，故善惊易惕，坐卧不安，恶闻声响；舌淡、苔黄滑腻，为气血亏虚，血不荣舌，痰湿内停之征；脉细略数或细弦为气虚血亏，心虚胆怯之象。

Syndrome analysis: the heart is the house of the mind, and heart qi deficiency causes insufficient nourishment of heart spirit, so appear palpitation, restlessness, insomnia, dreaminess and easy wake-up. Weakness and timidity of gallbladder qi leads to easy wake-up, restlessness and sensitivity to loud noise. Pale tongue with yellow slippery and greasy fur is the manifestation of internal retention of phlegm-dampness that is caused by qi and blood deficiency failing to nourish the tongue. Thready and slightly rapid pulse or thready wiry pulse suggests qi and blood deficiency and heart deficiency as well as gallbladder timidity.

2015 年 11 月 19 日二诊：精神佳，失眠症状好转，但仍有害怕，余无异常，舌淡，苔黄腻（图 3.2.1.5b），脉细。原方加珍珠母 30g，继续服用 7 剂，嘱注意休息，保持心情舒畅。

Second visit on November 19, 2015: the spirit and insomnia were improved, but he was still susceptible to fright, and other symptoms were normal. The tongue was pale with yellow-greasy fur (Fig.3.2.1.5b), and the pulse was thready. Seven doses of the previous prescription with the addition of zhenzhumu 30g were administered for further treatment. And the patient was advised to have good rest and be in a good mood.

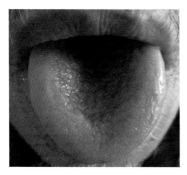 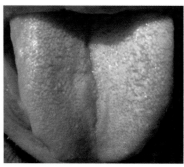

图 3.2.1.5a
Fig.3.2.1.5a

图 3.2.1.5b
Fig.3.2.1.5b

（六）心悸 – 湿热浸淫证

1.6 Palpitation: syndrome of dampness-heat intrusion and spreading

患者郑某，男，72 岁，反复胸闷、心慌 5 年余加重 1 月，于 2017 年 5 月 15 日就诊。

Patient Zheng, male, 72 years old, had been suffering from recurrent chest distress and flusteredness for more than 5 years, the symptoms aggravated one month ago and he visited the doctor on May 15, 2017.

患者有高血压病、冠状动脉粥样硬化性心脏病史，长期服用氯沙坦、氢氯噻嗪片，血压控制尚可。1 个月前患者胸闷、心慌等症状加重，遂来就诊。刻诊：胸闷，心慌，气短，活动后加重，头晕，晨起明显，伴视物旋转，无头痛，咳嗽咯痰，黄色黏痰，鼻塞流浊涕，双上肢不自主颤动，易出汗，纳食欠佳，易腹胀，夜寐欠佳，大便溏泄，小便可，舌质暗，苔黄腻（图 3.2.1.6a），脉弦滑。动态心电图示：窦性心动过速，心律不齐，一过性 T 波改变。心脏彩超示：左室舒张功能减退。

The patient had a history of hypertension and coronary atherosclerotic heart disease and has been taking losartan and hydrochlorothiazide tablets to control the hypertension with good effect. Chest distress and flusteredness aggravated one month ago, so he visited the doctor. Present symptoms: chest distress, flusteredness, shortness of breath that aggravates after activity, dizziness that is more obvious in the morning and accompanied with visual rotation, no headache, cough with expectoration of yellow sticky phlegm, nasal congestion with turbid snivel, involuntary tremor of upper limbs, easy sweating, poor appetite, easy abdominal distension, sleepless at night, loose stool, normal urine, dark purple tongue with yellow greasy fur (Fig.3.2.1.6a), and wiry slippery pulse. The dynamic electrocardiogram showed that sinus tachycardia, arrhythmia, and transient T-wave change. Cardiac color ultrasound showed that the left ventricular diastolic function decreased.

西医诊断：窦性心动过速，心律不齐。

Western medicine diagnosis: sinus tachycardia, arrhythmia.

中医诊断：心悸。

TCM diagnosis: palpitation.

辨证：湿热浸淫，气血不运证。

Syndrome differentiation: dampness-heat intrusion and spreading, transportation disorder of qi and blood.

治疗：清热化湿，宁心安神。

Treatment: clearing heat and resolving dampness, calming heart and tranquilizing mind.

处方：葛根黄芩黄连汤加减：葛根 10g，黄芩 10g，黄连 6g，石菖蒲 10g，茯苓 10g，郁金 10g，苦参 10g，板蓝根 10g，厚朴 10g，枳壳 10g，白扁豆 15g。10 剂，日 1 剂，水煎，分 2 次温服。

Prescription: modified *Gegen Huangqin Huanglian* Decoction.

Gegen 10g, huangqin 10g, huanglian 6g, shichangpu 10g, fuling 10g, yujin 10g, kushen 10g, banlangen 10g, houpo 10g, zhiqiao 10g, baibiandou 15g.

Ten doses and one dose a day, decoction, take twice warmly.

证候分析：湿热内蕴，阻碍气机，气机壅滞则胸闷、气短；湿热蕴酿于中焦，升降失司，可见纳食欠佳、腹胀；清阳不升则头晕，气机壅滞于肺，肺失宣降，可见咳嗽咯痰、鼻塞等症状；舌质紫暗，乃湿热阻止，血行不畅而成瘀；苔黄腻为湿热内蕴之征。

Syndrome analysis: internal accumulation of dampness-heat obstructs qi movement, which leads to chest distress and shortness of breath. Dampness-heat accumulating in the middle energizer causes the abnormal ascending and descending of qi, which results in poor appetite and abdominal distension. Lucid yang failing to rise triggers dizziness. Qi stagnation in the lung makes the failure of lung to depurate and descend, therefore, cough with expectoration, nasal congestion and other symptoms occur. The tongue is dark and purple, indicates internal heat-dampness, yellow-greasy fur indicates that dampness-heat accumulated. Dark purple tongue indicates the blood stasis caused by dampness-heat obstruction and unsmooth circulation of the blood, and yellow greasy fur is the main manifestation of internal accumulation of dampness-heat.

2017 年 5 月 22 日二诊：胸闷缓解，咳嗽减轻，大小便正常，舌淡紫、苔薄黄（图 3.2.1.6b），脉弦。原方减板蓝根，加薏苡仁 20g，7 剂，巩固治疗。

Second visit on 22 May, 2017: chest distress and cough were relieved, stool and urine were normal, the tongue turned pale purple with thin and yellow fur (Fig.3.2.1.6b), and the pulse was wiry. Seven doses of the previous prescription were administered to consolidate the effect, with the reduction of banlangen and the addition of yiyiren 20g.

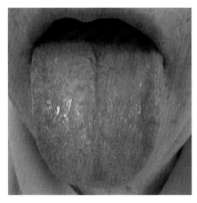 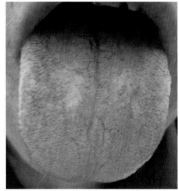

图 3.2.1.6a 图 3.2.1.6b
Fig.3.2.1.6a Fig.3.2.1.6b

（七）不寐 – 心脾两虚证

1.7 Insomnia: syndrome of dual deficiency of heart and spleen

患者唐某，女，42 岁，失眠 10 年加重 3 个月，于 2012 年 3 月 22 日就诊。

Patient Tang, female, 42 years old, had been suffering from insomnia for 10 years and the symptom aggravated 3 months ago. Then she came to visit the doctor on March 22, 2012.

患者 10 年前因行子宫切除术后出现失眠，经中西医治疗效果不甚明显，长期服用舒乐安定维持，近 3 个月来患者因劳累至失眠症状加重，遂来就诊。刻诊：精神疲倦，头晕、心悸，夜间入睡困难，时寐时醒，纳差，小便量多，大便秘结，3 ～ 5 日一行，舌暗淡，苔薄白（图 3.2.1.7a），脉细。

The patient had insomnia after the hysterectomy 10 years ago and was treated with Chinese and Western medicine with no obvious effect. The patient took estazolam to control the symptom for a long time. Insomnia aggravated in recent 3 months because of overwork, so she came for treatment. Present symptoms: fatigue, dizziness, palpitation, difficulty in falling asleep at night with easy wake-up, poor diet, profuse urine, dry stool with one defecation every 3-5 days, dark pale tongue with thin white fur (Fig.3.2.1.7a), and thready pulse.

西医诊断：神经症。

Western medicine diagnosis: neurosis.

中医诊断：不寐。

TCM diagnosis: insomnia.

辨证：心脾两虚，心神失养证。

Syndrome differentiation: dual deficiency of heart and spleen, insufficient nourishment of heart spirit.

治疗：健脾养心安神。

Treatment: invigorating spleen and nourishing heart and tranquilizing mind.

处方：归脾汤加减：党参 15g，黄芪 20g，茯神 20g，龙眼肉 15g，远志 10g，炒酸枣仁 20g，夜交藤 30g，合欢皮 20g，木香 6g，麦芽 15g，白术 15g，茯苓 15g，当归 12g，大枣 3 枚。7 剂，日 1 剂，水煎，分 2 次温服。

Prescription: modified *Guipi* Decoction.

Huangqi 20g, fushen 20g, longyanrou 15g, yuanzhi 10g, chaosuanzaoren 20g, yejiaoteng 30g, hehuanpi 20g, muxiang 6g, maiya 15g, baizhu 15g, fuling 15g, danggui 12g, dazao 3 pieces.

Seven doses and one dose a day, decoction, take twice warmly.

证候分析：脾虚运化功能失职，气血生化不足，血虚不能养心，则心悸、失眠；

气血不能上濡清窍，则头晕；脾虚运化水谷功能失职，则纳差；肢体失养，则倦怠乏力；舌暗淡、苔薄白，脉细，为心脾气血不足之象。

Syndrome analysis: spleen deficiency with dysfunction of transportation and transformation leads to the insufficiency generation of qi and blood, which cannot nourish the heart, so palpitation and insomnia occur. Qi and blood cannot nourish the lucid orifice, then dizziness appears. Spleen deficiency failing to transport and transform the essence of water and grain causes poor diet. Deficient cultivation of limbs and body leads to fatigue. Dark pale tongue with thin white fur and thready pulse are the signs of qi and blood deficiency of the heart and spleen.

2012 年 3 月 29 日二诊：服上药后睡眠症状改善明显，夜寐 5 小时左右，舌淡红、苔薄白（图 3.2.1.7b），脉缓。为巩固疗效，守上方继续服用。

Second visit on March 29, 2012: insomnia was improved significantly after medication. The patient could sleep 5 hours at night and had pale red tongue with thin white fur (Fig.3.2.1.7b) as well as moderate pulse. The previous prescription was used to consolidate the curative effect.

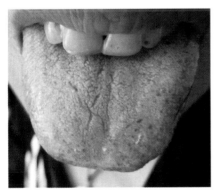 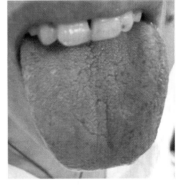

图 3.2.1.7a | 图 3.2.1.7b
Fig.3.2.1.7a | Fig.3.2.1.7b

（八）不寐－心肾不交证

1.8 Insomnia: syndrome of non-interaction between heart and kidney

患者吴某，男，63 岁，失眠 10 年加重半月，于 2014 年 7 月 15 日就诊。

Patient Wu, male, 63 years old, had been suffering from insomnia for 10 years and the symptom aggravated half a month ago. Then he came to visit the doctor on

June 15, 2014.

患者自诉失眠 10 余年，时轻时重，甚至通宵不寐，曾口服地西泮、中药等治疗，但失眠症状没有治愈。近日患者失眠症状加重，甚至通宵不寐，遂就诊。刻诊：形体消瘦，腰膝酸软，双口角生疮，头昏痛，口渴多饮，纳可，大便偏干，日 1 次，小便可，舌质紫红，少苔（图 3.2.1.8a），脉沉而细数。

The patient had been suffering from insomnia for more than 10 years with the symptom from mild to severe, or even insomnia all night. He was treated with diazepam and Chinese medicine orally, but the insomnia was not cured. Symptoms of insomnia had worsened recently, or even insomnia all night, so he came to see the doctor. Present symptoms: emaciation, soreness and weakness of the waist and knee, sores in the corners of the mouth, dizziness and headache, thirsty with desire to drinks, normal diet, dry stool with one defecation a day, normal urine, purple red tongue with little fur (Fig.3.2.1.8a), deep thready and rapid pulse.

西医诊断：神经症。

Western medicine diagnosis: neurosis.

中医诊断：不寐。

TCM diagnosis: insomnia.

辨证：心肾不交，水火不济证。

Syndrome differentiation: non-interaction between heart and kidney.

治疗：滋阴潜阳，交通心肾。

Treatment: nourishing yin and subduing yang, restoring coordination between heart and kidney.

处方：交泰丸加减：酸枣仁 15g，天麻 10g，熟地黄 15g，龟甲 20g（先煎），牡蛎 20g（先煎），黄连 3g，肉桂 1g（后下），川芎 3g。7 剂，日 1 剂，水煎，分 2 次温服。

Prescription: modified *Jiaotai* Pill.

Suanzaoren 15g, tianma 10g, shudihuang 15g, guijia 20g (decocted first), muli 20g (decocted first), huanglian 3g, rougui 1g (decocted later), chuanxiong 3g.

Seven doses and one dose a day, decoction, take twice warmly.

证候分析：肾水不足，不能上济心火，使心火偏旺，内扰心神，则失眠多梦；心火上蒸，则口角生疮，头昏痛，口渴多饮；心火下移，肾水亏虚，腰府失养，则腰膝酸软；舌质红，少苔，脉沉而细数，为阴不足而阳偏亢之象。

Syndrome analysis: insufficient kidney water cannot restrict the heart fire which makes the heart fire effulgent and disturbs the heart spirit, so insomnia and dreaminess occur. The heart fire flames upward which makes sores in the corners of the mouth, dizziness and headache, and thirsty with desire to drinks, meanwhile, the heart fire moves down which makes kidney water deficiency and insufficient nourishment of the waist, then appears weakness of the waist and knee. Red tongue with little fur and deep, thready and rapid pulse are the manifestations of yin deficiency and yang hyperactivity.

2014 年 7 月 22 日二诊：患者可夜寐 3 ～ 4 小时，口渴症状有所减轻，舌淡紫、苔薄（图 3.2.1.8b），脉细。继服上方 7 剂。后夜寐症状好转，通宵不寐之象消除。

Second visit on July 22, 2014: the patient could sleep 3-4 hours at night, with thirst alleviated, pale purple tongue with thin fur (Fig.3.2.1.8b), and thready pulse. Seven doses of the above prescription were administered. Then the sleep at night was further improved with insomnia all night eliminated.

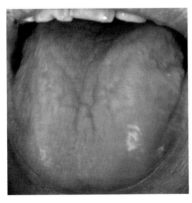 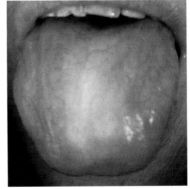

图 3.2.1.8a
Fig.3.2.1.8a

图 3.2.1.8b
Fig.3.2.1.8b

（九）胸痹 – 气滞血瘀证

1.9　Chest impediment: syndrome of qi stagnation and blood stasis

患者付某，女，60 岁，胸闷不适半年加重 1 周，于 2017 年 5 月 17 日就诊。

Patient Fu, female, 60 years old, had been suffering from chest distress for half a year and the symptom aggravated one week ago. Then she came to see the doctor on May 17, 2017.

患者半年前无明显诱因出现胸闷不适，未系统治疗。近 1 周来，患者胸闷不适症状加重，遂来就诊。刻诊：胸闷、胸痛，天气变化后加重，休息后可改善，平素性情急躁，两肋感胀满不适，伴头晕头痛，以两侧明显。视物模糊，步履欠稳，向左侧偏行，四肢肌力正常，口干，时有反酸嗳气，纳食尚可，夜寐可，大便干结，小便调。舌绛紫，苔黄腻（图 3.2.1.9a），脉沉细。心脏彩超示：左房轻度增大，左室舒张功能减退。胸部 CT 平扫示未见明显异常。心电图提示：窦性心动过缓，T 波轻度改变。

The patient suffered from chest distress six months ago without obvious cause and she wasn't treated systematically. The symptom aggravated one week ago, so she came to see the doctor. Present symptoms: chest distress and pain that aggravates with the weather change and alleviates with rest. She was short-tempered and felt distension and discomfort in hypochondrium, dizziness, headache (especially in laterals), blurred vision, unsteady steps that deviate to the left, normal myodynamia of the limbs, dry mouth, acid regurgitation and belching sometimes, normal diet and sleep, dry stool, normal urine, crimson purple tongue with yellow greasy fur (Fig.3.2.1.9a), deep and thready pulse. Cardiac color ultrasound: the left atrium slightly increased, the left ventricular diastolic function decreased. Chest CT scan showed no obvious abnormality. Electrocardiogram (ECG): sinus bradycardia, and T wave slightly changed.

西医诊断：冠状动脉粥样硬化性心脏病。

Western medicine diagnosis: coronary atherosclerotic heart disease.

中医诊断：胸痹。

TCM diagnosis: chest impediment.

辨证：气滞血瘀，心脉不畅证。

Syndrome differentiation: qi stagnation and blood stasis, heart vessel obstruction.

治疗：益气养阴，活血化瘀。

Treatment: replenishing qi and nourishing yin, activating blood and resolving stasis.

处方：生脉饮加减：党参 15g，麦冬 15g，五味子 5g，瓜蒌皮 15g，薤白 15g，法半夏 10g，水蛭 3g，降香 15g，山茱萸 15g，炙黄芪 20g，柴胡 10g，陈皮 10g，茯苓 15g，丝瓜络 10g，肉桂 2g，甘草 6g，黄连 6g，三七粉 3g（冲服），甘松 10g，红花 10g，石斛 10g。7 剂，日 1 剂，水煎，分 2 次温服。

Prescription: modified *ShengMai* Decoction.

Dangshen 15g, maidong 15g, Wuweizi 5g, gualoupi 15g, xiebai 15g, fabanxia 10g, shuizhi 15g, jiangxiang 15g, shanzhuyu 15g, zhihuangqi 20g, chaihu 10g, chenpi 10g, fuling 15g, sigualuo 10g, rougui 2g, gancao 6g, huanglian 6g, sanqifen 3g (take medicine with water), gansong 10g, honghua 10g, shihu 10g.

Seven doses and one dose a day, decoction, take twice warmly.

证候分析：气机阻滞，则出现胸闷，胀痛；脾失健运，运化失司，可见反酸嗳气；血脉不畅以致血瘀，筋脉失养，则步履不稳；气血蕴久化热，舌绛紫、苔黄腻提示瘀滞湿热内盛。

Syndrome analysis: qi movement blockage brings on chest distress and pain. Failure of the spleen to transport and transform leads to acid regurgitation and belching. Unsmooth blood circulation induces blood stasis and insufficient nourishment of sinews and vessels, so unsteady steps appear. The internal accumulation of qi and blood transforming into heat and crimson purple tongue with yellow greasy fur indicate blood stasis and internal excessive dampness-heat.

2017 年 5 月 24 日二诊：胸闷症状减轻，无胸痛，胁肋部无胀感，偶有反酸嗳气，二便可，舌紫红，苔黄（图 3.2.1.9b），脉濡。原方加代赭石 30g、海螵蛸 15g，7 剂，继续治疗。

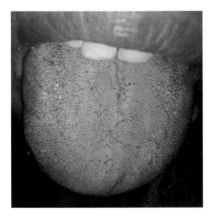
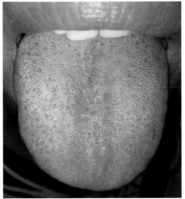

图 3.2.1.9a　　　　　　　　　图 3.2.1.9b
Fig.3.2.1.9a　　　　　　　　Fig.3.2.1.9b

Second visit on May 24, 2017: chest distress was relieved, and the patient had no chest pain, no distension in hypochondrium, acid regurgitation and belching sometimes, normal stool and urine, purple red tongue with yellow fur (Fig.3.2.1.9b), and soggy pulse. Seven doses of the previous prescription were administered for further treatment, with the addition of daizheshi 30g and haipiaoxiao 15g.

（十）胸痹 – 心脉瘀阻证

1.10　Chest impediment: syndrome of heart stasis obstruction

患者常某，女，37 岁，胸闷胸痛 7 年加重 3 天，于 2015 年 4 月 10 日就诊。

Patient Chang, female, 37 years old, had been suffering from chest distress and pain for 7 years and the symptoms aggravated 3 days ago. Then she came to visit the doctor on April 10, 2015.

患者 7 年前因胸闷时常发作，于某医院诊断为"冠状动脉粥样硬化性心脏病"，长期服降压、降脂、扩血管药物治疗。7 天前患者因劳累致胸闷胸痛症状加重遂来就诊。刻诊：形体肥胖，口唇发绀，左侧胸闷、胸痛，夜间为甚，痛处固定，拒按，无咳嗽、咯痰，纳可，寐差，二便正常，舌质暗有瘀斑，苔白腻（图 3.2.1.10a），脉弦涩。血压：150/110mmHg。心电图示：窦性心律，S-T 段压低、T 波低平。心脏彩超示：左心室肥厚。

The patient had been diagnosed "coronary atherosclerotic heart disease" with frequent chest distress 7 years ago in local hospital and treated with antihypertensive agents, lipid-lowering agents and blood vessel-dilating medicines. Seven days ago, the symptoms of chest distress and pain aggravated because of fatigue, so she came for treatment. Present symptoms: fat body, cyanotic lips, left chest distress and pain that aggravates at night with fixed position and is unpalpable, no cough, no expectoration, normal appetite, insomnia, normal urine and stool, dark tongue with ecchymosis and white greasy fur (Fig.3.2.1.10a), and wiry unsmooth pulse. Blood pressure: 150/110mmHg. Electrocardiogram: sinus rhythm, S-T segment depression, T wave flat. Cardiac color ultrasound: left ventricular hypertrophy.

西医诊断：冠状动脉粥样硬化性心脏病。

Western medicine diagnosis: coronary atherosclerotic heart disease.

中医诊断：胸痹。

TCM diagnosis: chest impediment.

辨证：心脉瘀阻，血行不畅证。

Syndrome differentiation: heart vessel stasis obstruction and blood circulation obstruction.

治疗：活血化瘀，通脉止痛。

Treatment: activating blood and resolving stasis, dredging vessel and relieving pain.

处方：血府逐瘀汤加减：丹参 15g，当归 10g，生地黄 10g，桃仁 10g，红花 10g，赤芍 12g，牛膝 20g，桔梗 10g，枳壳 10g，柴胡 8g，川芎 10g，瓜蒌 15g，甘草 5g。7 剂，日 1 剂，水煎，分 2 次温服。

Prescription: Modified *Xuefu Zhuyu* Decoction.

Danshen 15g, danggui 10g, shengdihuang 10g, taoren 10g, honghua 10g, chishao 12g, niuxi 20g, jiegeng 10g, zhiqiao 10g, chaihu 8g, chuanxiong 10g, gualou 15g, gancao 5g.

Seven doses and one dose a day, decoction, take twice warmly.

证候分析：血行瘀滞，胸阳痹阻，心脉不畅，不通则痛；夜间阳气虚衰，血流运行减缓，故心胸疼痛，痛有定处，入夜为甚；瘀血阻络，心脉失养，心神不宁则寐差；口唇发绀，舌质暗有瘀斑，苔白腻，脉弦涩，为心血瘀阻，气化失职之象。

Syndrome analysis: blood stagnancy and chest yang obstruction cause unsmooth heart vessel and chest pain. Yang qi is weak at nigh which makes the blood flowing slow down, so chest pain aggravates at night with fixed position. Blood stasis blocks collaterals, which causes insufficient nourishment of heart vessel and restlessness of heart spirit, so insomnia occurs. Cyanotic lips, dark tongue with ecchymosis, white greasy fur, and wiry unsmooth pulse are the signs of heart blood stagnancy and abnormal qi transformation.

2015 年 4 月 17 日二诊：胸闷、胸痛症状明显好转，睡眠转佳，余无不适，舌质暗红，苔白稍腻（图 3.2.1.10b），脉弦。嘱守前方继续服用。

Second visit on April 17, 2015: chest distress and pain were improved significantly, and the patient had better sleep, no other discomfort, dark red tongue with white and slightly greasy fur (Fig.3.2.1.10b), and wiry pulse. The above prescription was still used for further treatment.

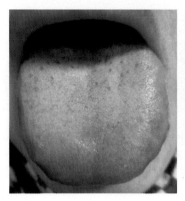 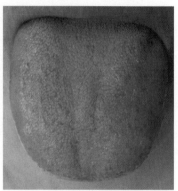

图 3.2.1.10a

Fig.3.2.1.10a

图 3.2.1.10b

Fig.3.2.1.10b

（十一）胸痹 – 痰瘀互结证

1.11　Chest impediment: syndrome of phlegm and stasis binding

患者毛某, 男, 62 岁, 反复胸闷心慌 10 余年加重 2 天, 于 2017 年 5 月 25 日就诊。

Patient Mao, male, 62 years old, had been suffering from recurrent chest distress and flusteredness for more than 10 years, and the symptoms aggravated 2 days ago, so he came to see the doctor on May 25, 2017.

患者有高血压病史 30 年, 服用硝苯地平缓释片, 血压控制一般。2 天前患者胸闷心慌症状加重, 遂来就诊。刻诊：胸闷心慌, 气短, 呼吸困难, 休息后可缓解, 周身乏力, 无头晕头痛、咯痰、色白质稀, 无汗, 无口干口苦, 纳差, 寐差梦多, 大便可, 小便频, 精神一般。舌质紫暗, 苔黄腻（图 3.2.1.11a）, 脉弦结代。心脏彩超示：左心增大, 二尖瓣微少量反流；室间隔轻度增厚, 左室收缩、舒张功能减退。

The patient had a history of hypertension for 30 years, taking nifedipine sustained-release tablets to control the blood pressure with little effect. Chest distress and flusteredness aggravated two days ago, so he visited the doctor. Present symptoms: chest distress, flusteredness, shortness of breath, dyspnea that alleviates after rest, general fatigue, no dizziness and headache, expectoration of white thin phlegm, no sweat, no dry mouth and bitter taste, poor appetite, insomnia and dreaminess, normal stool and frequent urine, common spirit state, dark purple tongue with yellow greasy fur (Fig.3.2.1.11a), wiry and regularly or irregularly intermittent pulse. Cardiac color ultrasound: the left heart enlarged and slight regurgitation of the mitral valve; the ventricular septum slightly thickened, and the left ventricular systolic and diastolic function decreased.

西医诊断：冠状动脉粥样硬化性心脏病。

Western medicine diagnosis: coronary atherosclerotic heart disease.

中医诊断：胸痹。

TCM diagnosis: chest impediment.

辨证：痰瘀互结，心脉不畅证。

Syndrome differentiation: phlegm and static binding, heart vessel obstruction.

治疗：活血化瘀，理气化痰。

Treatment: activating blood and resolving stasis, regulating qi and resolving phlegm.

处方：涤痰汤合血府逐瘀汤加减：当归 15g，赤芍 15g，川芎 10g，桃仁 10g，红花 10g，牛膝 15g，柴胡 10g，桔梗 10g，茯苓 15g，陈皮 15g，半夏 10g，薤白 10g，夜交藤 30g，合欢皮 20g。7 剂，日 1 剂，水煎，分 2 次温服。

Prescription: modified *Ditan* Decoction together with *Xuefu Zhuyu* Decoction.

Danggui 15g, chishao 15g, chuanxiong 10g, taoren 10g, honghua 10g, niuxi 15g, chaihu 10g, jiegeng 10g, chenpi 15g, banxia 10g, xiebai 10g, yejiaoteng 30g, hehuanpi 20g.

Seven doses and one dose a day, decoction, take twice warmly.

证候分析：脾虚，生化不足，肢体失养，则周身乏力；脾虚不能运化水湿则生痰，气血亏虚，运行无力则成瘀，痰瘀互结，痹阻心胸，气机运行不畅，则胸闷、气短；痰浊壅肺，肺宣发肃降功能失职，则咳嗽、咯痰、呼吸困难；痰瘀日久化热，扰乱心神，则失眠多梦；舌质紫暗为瘀血内阻，舌失荣养；舌苔黄腻，脉弦滑数，为痰热、瘀血内阻之征象。

Syndrome analysis: spleen deficiency with insufficiency of generation and transformation leads to insufficient nourishment of the limbs and body, so general fatigue occur. Spleen deficiency failing to transport and transform water-dampness generates phlegm, and qi-blood deficiency failing to propel the blood circulation produces stasis. When phlegm and stasis bind together and obstruct the heart and chest, qi movement is hindered, and chest distress and shortness of breath appear.

Turbid phlegm obstructing lung causes failure of lung to depurate and descent, so symptoms such as cough, expectoration and dyspnea manifest. The transformation of phlegm-stasis into heat disturbs heart spirit, so insomnia and dreaminess occur. Dark purple tongue is caused by internal obstruction of blood stasis and insufficient nourishment of the tongue. And yellow greasy fur and wiry, slippery and rapid pulse are manifestations of internal obstruction of phlegm-heat and blood stasis.

2017 年 6 月 2 日二诊：患者精神好转，胸闷、心慌症状稍减，咳嗽减轻，无痰，夜寐 5 ～ 6 小时，大小便可，舌暗红，苔薄黄（图 3.2.1.11b），脉弦。继续原方 7 剂。

Second visit on June 9,2017: the patient's spirit was improved. Chest distress and flusteredness were slightly alleviated, and the cough was relieved without phlegm. The patient could sleep for 5-6 hours, with normal stool and urine, dark red tongue with thin yellow fur (Fig.3.2.1.11b), and wiry pulse. Seven doses of the previous prescription were administered for treatment.

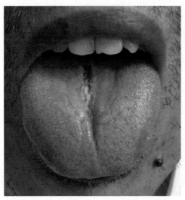 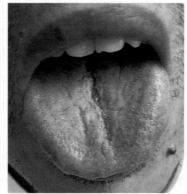

图 3.2.1.11a   图 3.2.1.11b
Fig.3.2.1.11a   Fig.3.2.1.11b

（十二）胸痹 – 痰瘀互结证

1.12 Chest impediment: syndrome of phlegm and stasis binding

患者万某，男，58 岁，胸闷、胸痛 1 年余加重 1 天，于 2017 年 5 月 11 日就诊。

Patient Wan, male, 58 years old, had been suffering from chest distress and pain for more than one year, and the symptoms aggravated one day ago. so he visited the doctor on May 11, 2017.

患者有高血压病史 4 余年，最高达 190/110mmHg，长期口服厄贝沙坦缓释片，血压控制欠佳，胸部闷痛 1 年余。1 天前患者因劳累后胸闷、胸痛症状加重，遂来就诊。刻诊：胸部闷痛，咳嗽，咯痰黄黏，无头晕头痛，无呕心呕吐，纳食可，夜寐梦多，大小便正常。舌质紫红，苔黄腻（图 3.2.1.12a），脉弦滑。动态心电图示：房性早搏，ST-T 改变。心脏彩超示：左房轻度增大，主动脉弹性降低。

The patient had a history of hypertension for more than 4 years, with a maximum of 190/110mmHg. He had been taking urbersartan sustained-release tablets orally for a long time without controlling well the blood pressure. He had been suffering from chest distress and pain for more than one year, and the symptoms aggravated due to overwork one day ago. So he visited the doctor. Present symptoms: chest distressand pain, cough with expectoration of yellow sticky phlegm, no dizziness and headache, no nausea and vomiting, normal appetite, dreamful sleep at night, normal stool and urine, purplered tongue with yellow greasy fur (Figure 3.2.1.12a), and wiry slippery pulse. Dynamic electrocardiogram: atrial premature beats, ST-T changed. Cardiac color ultrasound: the left atrial slightly enlarged and the aortic elasticity decreased.

西医诊断：冠心病。

Western medicine diagnosis: coronary heart disease.

中医诊断：胸痹。

TCM diagnosis: chest impediment.

辨证：痰瘀互结，心脉痹阻证。

Syndrome differentiation: phlegm and stasis binding, heart vessel obstruction.

治疗：活血化瘀，化痰通络。

Treatment: activating blood and resolving stasis, resolving phlegm and dredging collateral.

处方：涤痰汤合通窍活血汤加减：胆南星 6g，法半夏 6g，枳实 9g，茯苓 12g，陈皮 10g，石菖蒲 6g，竹茹 9g，白芷 10g，丹参 10g，赤芍 15g，桃仁 10g，川芎 10g，红花 10g，川牛膝 15g，生姜 3 片，大枣 6 枚。7 剂，日 1 剂，水煎，分 2 次温服。

Prescription: modified *Ditan* Decoction together with *Tongqiao Huoxue* Decoction.

Dannanxing 6g, fabanxia 6g, zhishi 9g, fuling 12g, chenpi 10g, shichangpu 6g, zhuru 9g, baizhi 10g, danshen 10g, chishao 15g, taoren 10g, chuanxiong 10g, honghua 10g, chuanniuxi 15g, shengjiang 3pieces, dazao 6 pieces.

Seven doses and one dose a day, decoction, take twice warmly.

证候分析：痰浊、瘀血互结，阻止心胸脉络，心脉失畅，则胸闷、胸痛；痰浊郁肺，肺失宣降，则咳嗽、咯痰；痰瘀日久化热，扰乱心神，则失眠多梦；舌紫红，苔黄腻，脉弦滑，为痰热内结，瘀阻化热之征。

Syndrome analysis: phlegm and stasis binding together obstructs the vessels and collaterals of the heart and chest, which causes insufficient nourishment of heart vessel and chest distress and pain. Phlegm turbidity depressing lung triggers failure of lung to depurate and descend, so cough and expectoration appear. The transformation of phlegm-stasis into heat disturbs heart spirit, so insomnia and dreaminess occur. Purplered tongue with yellow greasy fur and wiry slippery pulse are manifestations of internal binding of phlegm-heat and the transformation of stasis obstruction into heat.

2017 年 5 月 18 日二诊：胸闷、胸痛症状明显减轻，偶尔咳嗽，咳少量黄痰，余无不适，舌淡红，苔薄黄（图 3.2.1.12b），脉弦。原方加浙贝母 10g，7 剂，巩固治疗。

Second visit on May 18, 2017: the syndromes of chest distress and pain were obviously relieved. The patient occasionally coughed up scanty yellow phlegm and had no other discomfort, with pale red tongue, thin yellow fur (Fig.3.2.1.12b), and wiry pulse. Seven doses of the previous prescription were administered to consolidate the effect, with the addition of zhebeimu 10g.

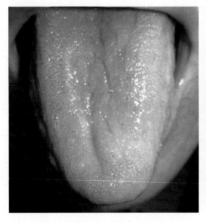 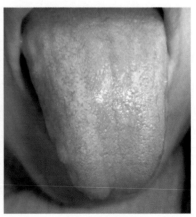

图 3.2.1.12a   图 3.2.1.12b

Fig.3.2.1.12a   Fig.3.2.1.12b

二、肝胆系病证

2. Liver and gallbladder system syndrome

（一）胁痛－肝胆湿热证

2.1 Hypochondriac pain: syndrome of dampness-heat in the liver and gallbladder

患者蔡某，男，54 岁，胁肋部胀痛伴口苦、口黏 1 月，于 2017 年 5 月 3 日就诊。

Patient Cai, male, 54 years old, had been suffering from distending pain in the hypochondrium with bitter taste and sticky feeling in the mouth for one month. So he visited the doctor on May 3,2017.

患者 1 个月以来自觉左侧胁肋部胀痛并伴口苦，口中黏腻，在家自行服药不能缓解，遂来就诊。刻诊：精神欠佳，四肢酸楚沉重，行走无力，面色潮红，语声高亢有力，自觉口中苦伴黏腻感，清晨起床时更明显，渴欲饮冷，纳可，偶有反酸，无嗳气，无恶心、呕吐，寐可梦多，小便平，大便黏滞不爽，日 1 次，舌质红，苔黄腻（图 3.2.2.1a），脉弦滑。腹部 B 超示：胆囊结石。

The patient had been feeling distending pain in the hypochondrium, accompanied with bitter taste and sticky feeling in the mouth for one month, and he visited the doctor after self-medication with little effect. Present symptoms: poor spirit, soreness and heaviness in limbs, forceless walking, flushed complexion, loud and powerful voice, bitter taste and sticky as well as greasy feeling in the mouth that aggravates especially in the morning get-up time, thirst with desire to cold drink, normal appetite, occasional acid regurgitation, no belching, no nausea or vomiting, dreamful sleep, normal urine, sticky stool with defecation once a day, red tongue with yellow greasy fur (Fig.3.2.2.1a), and wiry slippery pulse. Abdominal B ultrasound indicates: cholecystolithiasis.

西医诊断：胆囊结石。

Western medicine diagnosis: cholecystolithiasis.

中医诊断：胁痛。

TCM diagnosis: hypochondriac pain.

辨证：肝胆湿热证。

Syndrome differentiation: dampness-heat in the liver and gallbladder.

治疗：清热祛湿，疏利肝胆。

Treatment: clearing heat and removing dampness, soothing liver and disinhibiting gallbladder.

处方：甘露消毒丹加减：竹茹 15g，枳实 10g，陈皮 10g，白豆蔻 15g，藿香 10g（后下），茵陈 15g，滑石 10g，木通 10g，茯苓 15g，延胡索 15g，郁金 8g，黄芩 6g。7 剂，日 1 剂，水煎服。

Prescription: modified *Ganlu Xiaodu* Powder.

Zhuru 15g, zhishi 10g, chenpi 10g, baidoukou 15g, huoxiang 10g (decocted later), yinchen 15g, huashi 10g, mutong 10g, fuling 15g, yanhusuo 15g, yujin 8g, huangqin 6g.

Seven doses and one dose a day, decoction.

证候分析：湿热蕴结肝胆，肝胆疏泄不利，气机不畅，不通则通，可见胁肋部疼痛；热邪灼伤津液，则口渴、口苦、渴欲饮冷；湿热上蒸，则口中黏腻、面色潮红；湿性重浊黏滞，阻滞气机，则四肢酸楚沉重，行走无力、大便黏滞不爽；湿性阻滞气机，气血不运，则舌质红；苔薄黄腻，脉弦滑，为湿热内蕴之象。

Syndrome analysis: dampness-heat accumulating in liver and gallbladder affects the normal coursing function of the liver and gallbladder as well as qi movement, which eventually causes pain in the hypochondrium. Pathogenic heat consumes body fluid, which leads to thirst with desire to cold drink and bitter taste in the mouth. Up-steaming of dampness-heat causes sticky feeling in the mouth and flushed complexion. The heaviness and stickiness nature of dampness blocks qi movement, so the patient showed soreness and heaviness in limbs, forceless walking, and sticky stool. Dampness blocking qi movement causes qi and blood stagnation, so red tongue appears. Thin, yellow greasy fur and wiry slippery pulse indicate internal accumulation of dampness-heat.

2017 年 5 月 10 二诊：精神好转，胁肋部胀痛减轻，口中黏腻感减轻，无口苦，寐可，大便成形，日 1 次，舌质淡红，苔薄黄腻（图 3.2.2.1b），脉弦。维持原方，巩固疗效。

Second visit on May 10, 2017: the spirit was improved and the distending pain in the hypochondrium and sticky feeling in the mouth were also relieved. He felt no bitter taste in the mouth and had normal sleep, formed stool with defecation once a day, light red tongue with thin yellow and greasy fur (Fig.3.2.2.1b), and wiry pulse. The above prescription was still used to consolidate the efficacy.

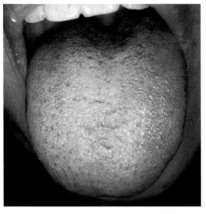

图 3.2.2.1a
Fig.3.2.2.1a

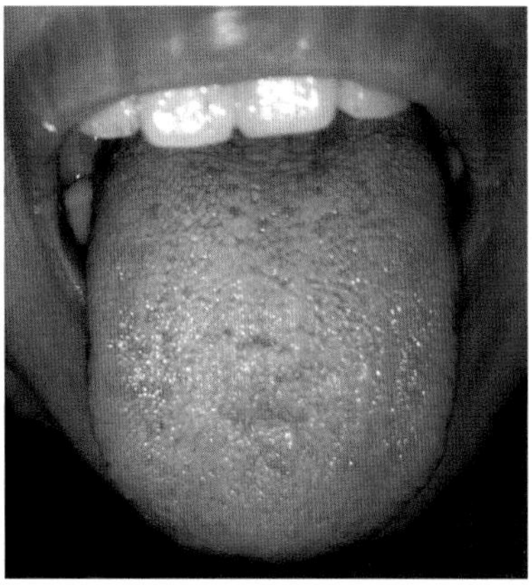

图 3.2.2.1b
Fig.3.2.2.1b

（二）胁痛 – 肝胆湿热证

2.2　Hypochondriac pain: syndrome of dampness-heat in the liver and gallbladder

患者汪某，男，51 岁，右胁胀痛 1 年余加重 1 月，于 2012 年 4 月 6 日就诊。

Patient Wang, male, 51 years old, had been suffering from distending pain in the right hypochondrium for more than one year and the symptom aggravated one month ago. Then he visited the doctor on April 6, 2012.

患者 1 年前因右胁胀痛而诊为乙型肝炎，间断服护肝、降脂药物治疗，1 月前右胁胀痛加重，遂来就诊。刻诊：肝区疼痛而胀、口苦口黏，耳胀头晕，纳差，精神疲乏，腰部酸痛，寐可梦多，小便短黄，大便日 1 次而不爽，舌质红，苔白腻夹黄（图 3.2.2.2a），脉弦滑。乙肝五项检查：乙型肝炎病毒表面抗原（＋），乙型肝炎病毒 e 抗原（＋），乙型肝炎病毒 e 抗体（＋）。肝功能：谷丙转氨酶 247U/L。

The patient was diagnosed as hepatitis B one year ago due to right hypochondriac pain, and he has been taking medicines for protecting the liver and lowering lipid intermittently. The symptom aggravated one month ago, so he came to visit the doctor. Present symptoms:distending pain in hepatic region, bitter taste with sticky feeling in the mouth, vertigo, distention in the ears, poor appetite, fatigue, aching pain in the waist, normal sleep with dreaminess, scanty brown urine, unsmooth defecation once a day, red tongue, white greasy and slightly yellow fur (Fig.3.2.2.2a), and wiry slippery pulse. Five tests for hepatitis B: HbsAg (+), HBeAg (+), HBeAb (+). Liver function test: ALT 247U/L.

西医诊断：乙型肝炎。

Western medicine diagnosis: hepatitis B.

中医诊断：胁痛。

TCM diagnosis: hypochondriac pain.

辨证：肝胆湿热证。

Syndrome differentiation: dampness-heat in the liver and gallbladder.

治疗：疏肝利胆，清热利湿。

Treatment: soothing liver and disinhibiting gallbladder, clearing heat and draining dampness.

处方：龙胆泻肝汤加减：龙胆 10g，柴胡 15g，栀子 10g，北沙参 15g，黄芩 10g，茵陈 15g，虎杖 10g，土茯苓 15g，白花蛇舌草 10g，金钱草 15g，车前草 10g，泽泻 10g，凤尾草 10g，炙甘草 5g。7 剂，日 1 剂，水煎服。

Prescription: modified *Longdan Xiegan* Decoction.

Longdan 10g, chaihu 15g, zhizi 10g, beishashen 15g, huangqin 10g, yinchen15g, huzhang10g, tufuling 15g, baihuasheshecao 10g, jinqiancao 15g, cheqiancao 10g, zexie 10g, fengweicao 10g, zhigancao 5g.

Seven doses and one dose a day, decoction.

证候分析：湿热蕴结肝经，肝络失和，疏泄失职，气机不畅，故右胁胀痛；肝为心之母，母病及子，内扰心神，则失眠多梦；肝为肾之子，子盗母气，影响及肾，则腰部酸痛；湿热下注，则小便短黄、大便不畅；湿热循肝胆经脉上移，则口苦口黏、耳胀头晕；舌质红，苔白腻夹黄，脉弦滑数，为肝胆湿热之象。

Syndrome analysis: dampness-heat accumulating in liver meridian causes the disharmony of liver collaterals, abnormal coursing function and qi movement blockage, which brings about distending pain in the right hypochondrium. Liver is the mother-organ of heart, whose disorder affects child-organ. Therefore, liver's disorder harasses heart spirit and results in insomnia and dreaminess. Liver is child-organ of kidney, whose disorder affects mother-organ. Therefore, liver's disorder involves in kidney and leads to aching pain in the waist. Downward flow of dampness-heat causes scanty brown urine and unsmooth defecation. Upward going of dampness along the liver and gallbladder meridians brings bitter taste with sticky feeling in the mouth, vertigo, and distention in the ears. Red tongue, white greasy and slightly yellow fur, and wiry slippery pulse are typical manifestations of dampness-heat in the liver and gallbladder.

2012 年 4 月 13 日二诊：肝区胀痛明显减轻，口不苦，小便清，纳可，舌质淡红，苔薄腻稍黄（图 3.2.2.2b），脉弦，守前方继续加减治疗，一月后复查肝功能：谷丙转氨酶 267U/L。继续以上方加减巩固治疗。

Second visit on April 13, 2012: distending pain in hepatic region was evidently alleviated without bitter taste, the urine was clear and the appetite was normal. The tongue was light red with thin greasy and slightly yellow fur (Fig.3.2.2.2b), and wiry pulse. Therefore, the previous prescription was still modified for treatment. The patient reexamined liver function one month later with the result of ALT 267U/ L. The previous prescription was still modified to consolidate the effect.

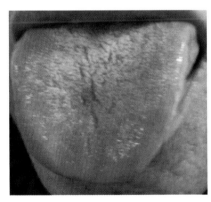 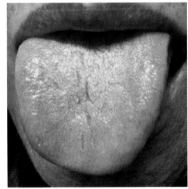

图 3.2.2.2a　　　　　　　　　图 3.2.2.2b
Fig.3.2.2.2a　　　　　　　　　Fig.3.2.2.2b

（三）胁胀 – 肝肾阴虚证

2.3 Hypochondriac pain: syndrome of yin deficiency of liver and kidney

患者范某，男，61 岁，肝功能异常 5 年，于 2017 年 3 月 29 日就诊。

Patient Fan, male, 61 years old, had been suffering abnormality in liver function for 5 years, so he visited the doctor on march 29, 2017.

患者 5 年前因胆石症行胆囊切除术时，查肝功能异常，长期服保肝护肝药物治疗，近来感觉左胁胀痛明显，遂来就诊。刻诊：精神体力不支，形体消瘦，时时耳鸣，面容憔悴、色白，左胁胀痛，口干、口苦，晨起明显，纳食无味，无反酸、嗳气，夜寐差、梦多，大便偏干，小便黄，舌质红，少苔（图 3.2.2.3a），脉弦细数。肝炎系列检查：（－）。腹部 B 超示：肝内胆管结石（较大者 12mm×8mm），脾大。上腹部 CT：肝内胆管结石并肝内胆管扩张，胆总管下段似见小结石，脾大，腹腔少量积液。

The patient had been found abnormality in liver function when experienced cholecystectomy for treating cholelithiasis 5 years ago, then he took a long period medication for protecting liver. Recently, the patient has felt distending pain in the left hypochondrium, therefore he visited the doctor. Present symptoms: poor mental and physical state, emaciation, frequent tinnitus, pale complexion with fatigue, distending pain in the left hypochondrium, dryness and bitterness in taste that aggravates in morning get-up time, reduced appetite without taste, no acid regurgitation and belching, poor sleep with dreaminess, dry stool and brown urine, red tongue with little fur (Fig.3.2.2.3a), and wiry thready rapid pulse. A series of hepatitis tests: (-).Abdominal B-mode ultrasound: intrahepatic bile duct stones (the bigger one about 12mm×8mm), splenomegaly. Epigastric CT: intrahepatic bile duct stones and expansion, with small stones in lower bile duct, splenomegaly, a small amount of hydrops in the abdomen.

西医诊断：乙型肝炎。

Western medicine diagnosis: hepatitis B.

中医诊断：胁胀。

TCM diagnosis: hypochondrium distention.

辨证：肝肾阴虚，肝络失养证。

Syndrome differentiation: yin deficiency of liver and kidney, insufficient nourishment of liver collaterals.

治疗：滋补肝肾，养阴柔络。

Treatment: nourishing liver and kidney, enriching yin and emolliating collaterals.

处方：一贯煎加减：北沙参 20g，生地黄 15g，麦冬 10g，瓜蒌子 15g，当归 10g，枸杞 10g，夜交藤 30g，酸枣仁 20g，川楝子 6g，地骨皮 10g。7 剂，日 1 剂，水煎服。

Prescription: modified *Yiguan* Decoction.

Beishasheng 20g, shengdihuang 15g, maidong 10g, gualouzi 15g, danggui 10g, gouqizi 10g, yejiaoteng 30g, suanzaoren 20g, chuanlianzi 6g, digupi 10g.

Seven doses and one dose a day, decoction.

证候分析：肝肾阴虚，虚热灼伤肝络，则胁肋部胀痛；阴虚，津液不能上承，则口干、口苦；阴虚，虚火内扰，则失眠、梦多；阴液亏虚，津液不能输布于大小肠，则大便干结、小便短黄；舌质红，少苔，脉弦细数，为阴虚内热之征象。

Syndrome analysis: yin deficiency of liver and kidney along with deficiency heat burns liver collaterals, which leads to the distending pain in left hypochondrium. Owing to yin deficiency, humor and fluid cannot spread upward which leads to dryness and bitterness in the mouth. Owing to yin deficiency, internal harassment of deficiency fire leads to insomnia and dreaminess. Yin deficiency with the failure of humor and fluid to distribute to small and large intestines causes dry stool and scanty brown urine. Red and thin tongue without fur and wiry thready rapid pulse are the manifestations of yin deficiency and internal heat.

2017 年 4 月 6 日二诊：精神好转，口干、口苦症状减轻，纳食乏味，左胁稍胀痛，寐可，小便清，大便软，日 1 次，舌淡红，苔薄黄（图 3.2.2.3b），脉弦细。原方减瓜蒌子 15g，加炒谷芽 15g、炒麦芽 15g、延胡索 15g、香附 6g，14 剂，继续治疗。

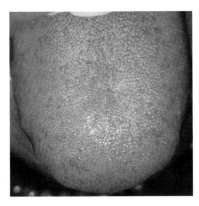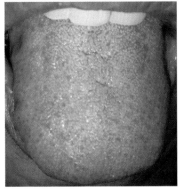

图 3.2.2.3a
Fig.3.2.2.3a

图 3.2.2.3b
Fig.3.2.2.3b

Second visit on April 6, 2017: the spirit was improvement, and dryness and bitterness in taste were relieved. The patient still had reduced appetite without taste, slight distending pain in the left hypochondrium,normal sleep, clear urine, soft stool with defecation once a day, light red tongue with thin yellow fur (Fig.3.2.2.3b), and wiry thready pulse. Fourteen doses of the previous prescription were administered for further treatment, with the reduction of gualouren and the addition of fried guya 15g, fried maiya 15g, yanhusuo 15g, and xiangfu 6g.

（四）胁胀 – 肝胆湿热证

2.4 Hypochondriac distention: syndrome of dampness-heat in the liver and gallbladder

患者王某，女，42 岁，乙肝 10 余年胁胀 10 天，于 2017 年 3 月 1 日就诊。

Patient wang, female, 42 years old, had been suffering from hepatitis B for more than 10 years. She felt hypochondriac distention 10 days ago, and then visited the doctor on May 1, 2017.

患者乙肝 10 余年，间断服保肝护肝药物治疗，近 10 日来，因纳食不慎致胁肋胀满不适，遂来就诊。刻诊：精力体力欠佳，面色黄，白睛黄染，食欲不振，厌油腻，食量少，食后脘痞不舒，时有胁肋部胀痛不适，情志不遂时加重，无恶心、呕吐、呃逆，舌质淡红，苔黄厚腻水滑（图 3.2.2.4a），脉弦数。乙肝六项示：乙型肝炎病毒表面抗原（+），乙型肝炎病毒 e 抗体（+），乙型肝炎病毒核心抗体（+），乙型肝炎病毒脱氧核糖核酸（–）。

The patient had been suffering from hepatitis B for more than 10 years with intermittent medication of liver-protecting drugs. She got hypochondriac distention and fullness for improper diet ten days ago, therefore she visited the doctor. Present symptoms: poor mental and physical state, yellow complexion and sclera, loss of appetite with reduced intake, dislike for greasy food, epigastric fullness and discomfort after eating, frequent distending pain in the hypochondrium that aggravated with bad emotion, no nausea, vomiting and hiccup, light red tongue with yellow, thick, greasy, watery and slippery fur (Fig.3.2.2.4a), and wiry rapid pulse. Six tests of hepatitis B: HBsAg (+), HBeAb (+), HBcAb (+), HBV-DNA (-).

西医诊断：乙型肝炎。

Western medicine diagnosis: hepatitis B.

中医诊断：胁胀。

TCM diagnosis: hypochondriac distention.

辨证：肝胆湿热证。

Syndrome differentiation: dampness-heat in the liver and gallbladder.

治疗：疏肝利胆，清热利湿。

Treatment: soothing liver and disinhibiting gallbladder, clearing heat and draining dampness.

处方：龙胆泻肝汤加减：栀子 10g，黄芩 10g，柴胡 10g，龙胆 15g，生地黄 10g，车前子 12g，泽泻 10g，茵陈 15g（后下），鸡内金 10g，厚朴 10g，枳壳 10g，郁金 10g。7 剂，日 1 剂，水煎服。

Prescription: modified *Longdan Xiegan* Decoction.

Zhizi 10g, huangqin 10g, chaihu 10g, longdan 15g, shengdihuang 10g, cheqianzi 12g, zexie 10g, yinchen 15g (decocted later), jineijin 10g, houpo 10g, zhiqiao 10g, yujin 10g.

Seven doses and one dose a day, decoction.

证候分析：湿热内蕴中焦，熏蒸肝胆，致胆汁外溢，则面黄、白睛黄染；湿热中阻，脾胃升降失职，则食欲不振，食量少；食后气机阻滞益甚，则脘痞不舒加重；湿热阻滞肝胆，气机不畅，则胁肋部胀痛不适；舌质淡红，苔黄厚腻，脉弦数，为湿热内阻之象。

Syndrome analysis: internal accumulation of dampness-heat in the middle energizer fumigates the liver and gallbladder, which causes the bile to overflow and results in yellow complexion and sclera. Dampness-heat blocking the middle energizer and dysfunction of spleen and stomach bring about loss of appetite with reduced intake. Increasing qi stagnation after eating aggravates epigastric fullness and discomfort. Dampness-heat blocking liver and gallbladder and qi stagnation cause distending pain in the hypochondrium. Light red tongue with yellow, thick, greasy fur and wiry rapid pulse are manifestations of internal blockage of dampness-heat.

2017 年 3 月 8 日二诊：目睛黄染已退，胁肋部胀痛减轻，纳少，二便正常，舌质淡红、苔薄黄根腻（图 3.2.2.4b），脉弦。原方减龙胆、栀子，加紫苏梗 10g、麦芽 15g、谷芽 15g，7 剂，继续治疗。

Second visit on March 8, 2017: yellow sclera was abated and distending pain in the hypochondrium was relieved. The patient had poor appetite, normal urine and stool, light red tongue with thin yellow fur and greasy tongue root (Fig.3.2.2.4b), and wiry pulse. Seven doses of the previous prescription were administered for further treatment, with the reduction of longdan, zhizi and the addition of zisugeng 10g, maiya 15g, and guya 15g.

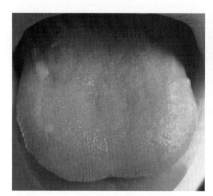
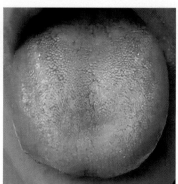

图 3.2.2.4a
Fig.3.2.2.4a

图 3.2.2.4b
Fig.3.2.2.4b

（五）奔豚气－肝郁气滞证

2.5　Running piglet qi: syndrome of liver depression and qi stagnation

患者谢某,女,29 岁,自觉气从少腹上冲至胸咽部 3 日,于 2014 年 3 月 10 日就诊。

Patient Xie, female, 29 years old, had suffered from adverse-rising qi from lower abdomen to chest and pharynx for 3 days, then she visited the doctor on March 10, 2014.

患者 3 天前与人发生争吵后,感觉两胁肋部胀闷不适,嗳气,之后感觉有一股气从少腹上冲胸咽部位,遂来就诊。刻诊：焦虑貌,精神紧张,自觉气从少腹上冲胸咽,时时嗳气,无恶心、呕吐,纳差,心悸失眠,两胁胀闷,二便可,舌质红,苔黄而干（图 3.2.2.5）,脉弦数。

After a quarrel 3 days ago, the patient felt distension and stuffiness in the hypochondrium, belching, and incontrollable adverse-rising qi from lower abdomen to chest and pharynx, so she visited the doctor. Present symptoms: anxious appearance, nervousness, adverse-rising qi from lower abdomen to chest and pharynx, frequent belching, no nausea and vomiting, poor appetite, palpitation and insomnia, distension and stuffiness in the hypochondrium, normal urine and stool, red tongue with yellow dry fur (Fig.3.2.2.5a), and wiry rapid pulse.

西医诊断：神经症。

Western medicine diagnosis: neurosis.

中医诊断：奔豚气。

TCM diagnosis: running piglet qi.

辨证：肝气不调，气机上逆证。

Syndrome differentiation: disharmony of liver qi, adverse-rising of qi movement.

治疗：平肝降逆，理气和胃。

Treatment: pacifying liver and descending adverse qi, regulating qi and harmonizing stomach.

处方：葛根芩连汤合酸枣仁汤加减：葛根 15g，黄芩 10g，白芍 15g，青皮 10g，川芎 10g，法半夏 10g，茯苓 15g，枳壳 10g，厚朴 10g，丁香 6g，龙齿 30g（先煎），酸枣仁 20g，生姜 5 片，甘草 3g。7 剂，日 1 剂，水煎服。

Prescription: modified *Gegen Qinlian* Decoction together with *Suanzaoren* Decoction.

Gegen 15g, huangqin 10g, baishao 15g, qingpi 10g, chuanxiong 10g, fabanxia 10g, fuling 15g, zhiqiao 10g, houpo 10g, dingxiang 6g, longchi 30g (decocted first), suanzaoren 20g, shengjiang 5 pieces, gancao 3g.

Seven doses and one dose a day, decoction.

证候分析：情志刺激，肝气郁结，气郁化火，气火随冲气上逆，则见气从少腹上冲胸咽；肝气郁结，气机不畅，则两胁胀闷；肝气横逆犯胃，胃失和降，则见嗳气、纳差；气火上扰心神，则心悸失眠；舌质红，苔黄而干，脉弦数，则为气郁化火之象。

Syndrome analysis: emotional stimulation causes liver qi depression that transforms into fire. Both qi and fire rises upward, therefore, the patient had adverse-rising qi from lower abdomen to chest and pharynx. Liver qi depression and qi movement inhibition triggers distension and stuffiness in the hypochondrium. Liver qi transversely attacks the stomach that causes the disharmony of stomach, therefore, the patient had belching and poor appetite.

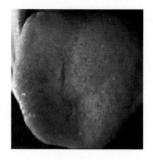

图 3.2.2.5
Fig.3.2.2.5

Upward harassment of qi and fire to heart spirit induces palpitation and insomnia. Red tongue with yellow dry fur and wiry rapid pulse are manifestations of depressed qi transforming into fire.

患者电话随访：患者诸症若失，病情痊愈。

Telephone follow-up showed that the patient had recovered with all the symptoms removed.

（六）积聚 – 湿热蕴结证

2.6 Abdominal mass: syndrome of dampness-heat accumulation

患者吴某，女，58 岁，右胁肋胀痛 10 余年加重 1 月，于 2016 年 3 月 5 日就诊。

Patient Wu, female, 58 years old, had been suffering from distending pain in the right hypochondrium for more than 10 years and the symptom aggravated one month ago. Then she visited the doctor on March 5, 2016.

患者脂肪肝史 10 余年，自我养生保健、服降脂茶等调理，但右胁时有疼痛。近 1 月来，患者因过食肥甘厚味而致右胁肋胀痛加重，遂来就诊。刻诊：面色潮红，右 胁肋胀痛、拒按，口干口渴、喜冷饮，烦躁易怒，易汗出，纳差，乏力，周身困重，小便黄，大便干，舌质紫暗，舌下络脉迂曲，苔黄厚腻（图 3.2.2.6a），脉弦滑数。

The patient had fatty liver for more than 10 years and takes lipid-lowering tea for healthcare, sometimes with pain in the right hypochondrium. The symptom aggravated one month ago because of over-eating fatty, greasy and sweet food in recent one month, so she visited the doctor. Present symptoms: tidal reddening of the face, unpalpable distending pain in the right hypochondrium, dry mouth and thirst with preference for cold drink, restlessness and irritability, easy sweating, poor appetite, fatigue, general heaviness, yellow urine, dry stool, dark purple tongue with yellow thick and greasy fur (Fig.3.2.2.6a), tortuous sublingual vessels, wiry slippery and rapid pulse.

西医诊断：脂肪肝。

Western medicine diagnosis: fatty liver.

中医诊断：积聚。

TCM diagnosis: abdominal mass.

辨证：肝脾不调，湿热蕴结证。

Syndrome differentiation: liver-spleen disharmony and internal accumulation of dampness-heat.

治疗：清热利湿、化痰祛瘀，调理肝脾。

Treatment: clearing heat and draining dampness, resolving phlegm and removing stasis, regulating liver and spleen.

处方：化肝煎加减：夏枯草 10g，丹参 15g，赤芍 10g，牡丹皮 15g，决明子 15g，火麻仁 15g，郁金 10g，柴胡 6g，香附 6g，虎杖 15g，泽泻 10g，炒薏苡仁 15g，鸡内金 10g，泽兰 10g，山楂 10g。7 剂，日 1 剂，水煎服。

Prescription: modified *Huagan* Decoction.

Xiakucao 10g, danshen 15g, chishao 10g, mudanpi 15g, juemingzi 15g, huomaren 15g, yujin 10g, chaihu 6g, xiangfu 6g, huzhang 15g, zexie 10g, chaoyiyiren 15g, jineijin 10g, zelan 10g, shanzha 10g.

Seven doses, and one dose a day, decoction.

证候分析：湿热困阻中焦脾胃，脾失健运，则纳差；聚湿成痰，阻止气机，则乏力、周身困重；湿热内蕴肝胆，胆郁痰扰，则烦躁易怒；痰热内扰，蒸津耗液，则汗出、口渴喜冷饮；湿热下注，则小便黄、大便干；热伤阴血，血行艰涩而成瘀，则舌质紫暗；苔黄厚腻，脉弦滑数，为湿热内蕴之象。

Syndrome analysis: dampness-heat accumulating in the middle energizer causes dysfunction of spleen in transportation and transformation, which brings about poor appetite. Dampness accumulation into phlegm hinders qi movement, which causes fatigue and general heaviness. Dampness-heat accumulating in liver and gallbladder causes gallbladder depression and phlegm harassment, which causes restlessness and irritability. Internal harassment of phlegm-heat steams body fluid, which leads to easy sweating, and thirst with preference for cold drink. Downward flow of dampness-heat brings about yellow urine and dry stool. Heat injuring yin blood makes difficult unsmooth circulation of the blood and blood stasis, therefore, dark purple tongue can be seen. Yellow thick and greasy fur and wiry slippery and rapid pulse indicate internal accumulation of dampness-heat.

2016 年 3 月 12 日二诊：右胁肋胀痛明显减轻，无口干、口苦，小便清，大便正常，日 1 次，仍有汗出，纳差，舌质淡紫，苔薄黄腻（图 3.2.2.6b），脉弦细。

原方减决明子、火麻仁，加瘪桃干 10g、浮小麦 20g、谷芽 15g、麦芽 15g。7 剂。嘱清淡饮食，调畅情志。

Second visit on March 12, 2016: pain in the right hypochondrium was significantly reduced and dry mouth and bitter taste were disappeared. The patient had clear urine, normal stool with defecation once a day, sweating, poor appetite, pale purple tongue with thin yellow and greasy fur(Fig.3.2.2.6b), and wiry thready pulse. Seven doses of the previous prescription were used for treatment with the reduction of juemingzi and huomaren and the addition of bietaogan 10g, fuxiaomai 20g, guya 15g, and maiya15g. The patient was asked to keep light diet and good mood.

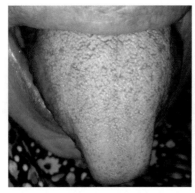 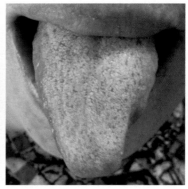

图 3.2.2.6a　　　　　　　　　图 3.2.2.6b
Fig.3.2.2.6a　　　　　　　　Fig.3.2.2.6b

（七）臌胀 – 水湿困脾证

2.7　Tympanites: syndrome of water-dampness encumbering spleen

患者刘某，男，57 岁，脘腹胀满半年加重 2 月，于 2015 年 5 月 15 日就诊。

Patient Liu, male, 57 years old, had been suffering from epigastric and abdominal distention and fullness for half a year and the symptoms aggravated 2 months ago. Then he visited the doctor on May 15, 2015.

患者半年前自觉脘腹胀满，食后胀满较甚，于当地医院就诊，查肝功能异常，诊断为"肝硬化腹水"，后多次行中、西医治疗，症状不减。近 2 月来，患者因劳累过度，腹胀症状加重，遂来就诊。刻诊：面色萎黄，形体消瘦，精神差，颜面、四肢轻度浮肿，腹部胀大，按之有振水音，纳差，寐差，不能平卧，小便短少，大便溏，舌质淡，苔白厚腻（图 3.2.2.7a），脉沉细。

When the patient went to local hospital half a year ago for epigastric and abdominal distention and fullness that aggravated after eating, he was diagnosed as abnormal liver function and ascites due to cirrhosis. Later he was treated with both Chinese and Western medicine for several times without obvious effect. He visited the doctor due to the aggravated abdominal distention in recent 2 months. Present symptoms: sallow complexion, emaciation, dispiritedness, mild edema of the face and limbs, enlarged abdomen with splashing sound when it is pressed, poor appetite, poor sleep, inability to lie flat, scanty urine, loose stool, pale tongue with white thick and greasy fur (Fig.3.2.2.7a), and deep thready pulse.

西医诊断：肝硬化腹水。

Western medicine diagnosis: ascites due to cirrhosis.

中医诊断：臌胀。

TCM diagnosis: tympanites.

辨证：肝脾不调证。

Syndrome differentiation: liver-spleen disharmony.

治疗：调肝理脾，温阳理气行水。

Treatment: regulating liver and spleen, warming yang, regulating qi and excreting water.

处方：胃苓汤合附子理中汤加减：党参 15g，炒白术 15g，茯苓 15g，猪苓 15g，泽泻 10g，大腹皮 10g，厚朴 10g，山楂 10g，夜交藤 20g，干姜 3g，附子 6g（先煎 1），怀山药 15g，陈皮 6g，木香 6g。7 剂，日 1 剂，水煎服。

Prescription: modified *Weiling* Decoction together with *Fuzi Lizhong* Decoction. Dangshen 15g, chaobaizhu 15g, fuling 15g, zhuling 15g, zexie 10g, dafupi 10g, houpo 10g, shanzha 10g, yejiaoteng 20g, ganjiang 3g, fuzi 6g (decocted first), huaishanyao 15g, chenpi 6g, muxiang 6g.

Seven doses and one dose a day, decoction.

证候分析：患者久病不愈，加之劳累过度，正气耗损，脾阳不振，水湿内停，蓄而不行，则腹大胀满，按之有水；中焦运化失职，则食后腹胀更甚，大便溏泻；脾病日久，气血生化不足，则形体消瘦，面色萎黄，神疲乏力；水湿困阻脾阳日久，影响及肾，致肾蒸化水液功能失常，则小便短少；水无出路，外溢肌肤，则颜面、四肢浮肿；舌苔白腻，脉沉细，为水湿内盛，中阳不振之象。

Syndrome analysis: the patient's prolonged illness and overstrain consumes healthy qi and causes hypofunction of the spleen and internal retention of water-dampness, therefore, there are abdominal distention and fullness, enlarged abdomen with splashing sound when it is pressed. Failure of the middle energizer to transport and transform causes loose stool and abdominal distention that aggravated after eating. Chronic disease of the spleen results in insufficient generation and transformation of qi and blood, which leads to sallow complexion, emaciation, dispiritedness and fatigue. Water-dampness encumbering spleen-yang affects the kidney's function of qi transformation, therefore, there is scanty urine. On the other hand, there is no outlet for water-dampness that overfalls to the muscle and skin, therefore, mild edema of the face and limbs appear. White greasy fur and deep thready pulse are manifestations of internal exuberance of water-dampness and devitalized middle yang.

2015 年 5 月 22 日二诊：精神较前好转，腹胀较前减轻，舌质淡，苔白腻（图 3.2.2.7b），脉沉。守方继续服用。

Second visit on May 22, 2015: the spirit was bettered and abdominal distention was alleviated. The tongue was pale with white greasy fur (Fig.3.2.2.7b), and the pulse was deep. The previous prescription was still used to consolidate the effect.

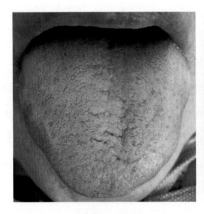 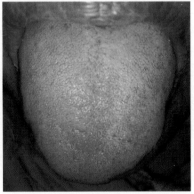

图 3.2.2.7a   图 3.2.2.7b
Fig.3.2.2.7a   Fig.3.2.2.7b

（八）郁证 – 肝郁气滞证

2.8　Depression: syndrome of liver depression and qi stagnation

患者孙某，女，58 岁，精神抑郁、焦虑不安 10 余年，于 2015 年 11 月 16 日就诊。

Patient Sun, female, 58 years old, had been suffering from mental depression and anxiety for more than 10 years. Then she visited the doctor on November 16, 2015.

患者长期以来情绪不稳，时有烦躁、焦虑，为求进一步治疗而就诊。刻诊：表情抑郁，情绪不稳，烦躁、焦虑，胁肋部胀满，周身燥热伴阵发性汗出，突发突止，寐差，口干，纳差，舌质红，苔白稍腻（图 3.2.2.8a），脉弦滑。胃镜检查示：非萎缩性胃炎。结肠镜检示：乙状结肠息肉，升结肠多发憩室。颈椎 MRI 示：颈椎病 I 型，T$_2$ 椎体血管瘤可能。咽喉镜检查示：咽喉炎。

The patient had been in mental disorder for a long time and sometimes accompanied with irritability and anxiety. In order to get a further treatment, she went to see the doctor. Present symptoms: depressed expression, emotional instability, irritability, anxiety, distention and fullness in the hypochondrium, general dryness-heat with paroxysmal sweating, poor sleep, dry mouth, poor appetite, red tongue with white and slightly greasy fur (Fig.3.2.2.8a), and wiry slippery pulse. Gastroscopy: non-atrophic gastritis. Colonoscopy: sigmoid polyp, multiple diverticulum in ascending colon. Cervical vertebral MRI: cervical spondylosis type I, T$_2$ vertebral hemangioma (possible). Laryngoscopy: laryngopharyngitis.

西医诊断：非萎缩性胃炎。

Western medicine diagnosis: non-atrophic gastritis.

中医诊断：郁证。

TCM diagnosis: depression syndrome.

辨证：肝郁气滞证。

Syndrome differentiation: liver depression and qi stagnation.

治疗：疏肝解郁，调畅情志。

Treatment: soothing liver and relieving depression, regulating emotion.

处方：柴胡疏肝散加减：柴胡 15g，当归 10g，白芍 15g，香附 8g，绿萼梅 10g，郁金 10g，茯苓 15g，夜交藤 30g，北沙参 15g，麦芽 15g，薄荷 6g（后下）。7 剂，日 1 剂，水煎服。

Prescription: modified *Chaihu Shugan* Powder.

Chaihu 15g, danggui 10g, baishao 15g, xiangfu 8g, lüemei 10g, yujin 10g, fuling 15g, yejiaoteng 30g, beishashen 15g, maiya 15g, bohe 6g (decocted later).

Seven doses and one dose a day, decoction.

证候分析：肝主气机，调畅情志。长期精神抑郁，情志不舒，致肝气郁滞，则胁肋部胀满；肝郁日久化火，迫津外泄，则周身燥热、汗出；肝火扰乱心神，则失眠；肝火犯胃，胃失和降，则口干，纳差；舌质红伴瘀点，为肝郁化火耗伤津血，致瘀之象；苔黄腻，为肝气郁结，气机不畅，水津不化之征；脉弦滑，为肝郁气滞之明证。

Syndrome analysis: the liver governs qi movement and regulates emotion. Long-term mental depression leads to liver qi depression and stagnation, which eventually results in distension and fullness in the hypochondrium; prolonged liver qi depression transforms into fire and causes body fluid to flow out, which leads to general dryness-heat with paroxysmal sweating; liver fire disturbing the heart spirit causes insomnia; liver fire attacking stomach makes stomach qi fail to descend and causes dry mouth and poor appetite. Liver qi depression transforms into fire and damages body fluid, leading to blood stasis with the presentation of red tongue with petechiae; yellow greasy fur is the manifestation of liver qi depression, unsmooth qi movement and failure of transformation of water and body fluid; wiry and slippery pulse is the typical manifestation of liver depression and qi stagnation.

2015 年 11 月 23 日二诊：情绪稳定，胁肋胀满症状减轻，仍烦躁，汗出，口干症状减轻，寐差，易惊醒，舌质淡红，苔白（图 3.2.2.8b），脉弦。原方加龙齿 30g、浮小麦 30g、煅龙骨 30g、煅牡蛎 30g，14 剂，继续治疗。逍遥丸调理善后。

Second visit on November 23, 2015: the patient was emotionally stable with relieved distention and fullness in the hypochondrium and dry mouth alleviated, but there were still irritability and sweating. The patient had poor sleep, easy wake-up, light red tongue with white fur (Fig.3.2.2.8b), and wiry pulse. Fourteen doses of the previous prescription were used for treatment, with the addition of longchi 30g, fuxiaomai 30g, duanlonggu 30g, and duanmuli 30g. *Xiaoyao* Pill was used for rehabilitation.

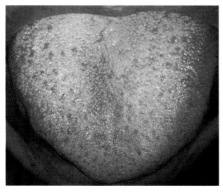 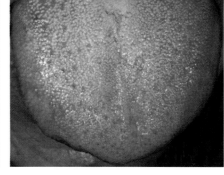

图 3.2.2.8a
Fig.3.2.2.8a

图 3.2.2.8b
Fig.3.2.2.8b

（九）黄疸 – 热重于湿证

2.9　Jaundice: syndrome of predominance of heat over dampness

患者郭某，男，64 岁，因突发皮肤及巩膜黄染 1 天，于 2011 年 8 月 11 日就诊。

Patient Guo, male, 64 years old, had sudden yellowed skin and sclera for one day, and he visited the doctor on August 11, 2011.

患者 1 天前不明原因出现皮肤及巩膜皆黄，急来就诊。刻诊：目睛、巩膜及皮肤全黄染，黄色鲜明如橘色，头晕，口苦口渴，脘腹胀满，呕恶纳呆，神疲乏力，倦怠嗜睡，午后发热，小便短赤，大便干结，舌质红，舌苔根部黄厚腻（图 3.2.2.9a），脉弦滑数。肝功能示：谷丙转氨酶 257U/L，谷草转氨酶 891U/L，碱性磷酸酶 187U/L，谷氨酸转移酶 124U/L，直接胆红素 6.3 μmol/L，间接胆红素 19 μmol/L。

The patient had sudden yellowed skin and sclera one day ago with unknown reasons, and hurried to visit the doctor. Present symptoms: eye, sclera and skin were all as bright yellow as orange. He felt dizzy, bitter taste in the mouth and thirst, abdominal fullness and distention, nausea, vomiting, anorexia, dispiritedness, lassitude, sleepiness, fever in the afternoon, scanty and dark urine, dry stool, red tongue with yellow, thick and greasy fur at its root(Fig.3.2.2.9a), wiry,slippery and rapid pulse. Liver function: ALT 257U/L, AST 891U/L, ALP 187U/L, GGT 124U/L, DBIL 6.3 μmol/L, IBIL 19 μmol/L.

西医诊断：急性黄疸型肝炎。

Western medicine diagnosis: acute icteric hepatitis.

中医诊断：黄疸。

TCM diagnosis: jaundice.

辨证：肝失疏泄，湿热内蕴证。

Syndrome differentiation: dysfunction of the liver in governing free flow of qi, internal accumulation of dampness-heat.

治疗：疏肝利胆退黄。

Treatment: soothing liver, disinhibiting gallbladder, and abating jaundice.

处方：茵陈蒿汤加减：茵陈 30g，柴胡 10g，黄芩 10g，栀子 10g，陈皮 10g，法半夏 10g，苍术 10g，厚朴 15g，竹茹 15g，凤尾草 15g，生大黄 6g（后下）。7 剂，日 1 剂，水煎服。

Prescription: modified *Yinchenhao* Decoction.

Yinchen 30g, chaihu 10g, huangqin 10g, zhizi 10g, chenpi 10g, fabanxia 10g, cangzhu 10g, houpo 15g, zhuru 15g, fengweicao 15g, shengdahuang 6g (decocted later).

Seven doses and one dose a day, decoction.

证候分析：湿热内蕴中焦，熏蒸肝胆，致胆汁外溢，故身目俱黄；热为阳邪，故黄色鲜明如橘色；热灼伤津，阳明燥结，故发热口渴，小便短赤，大便秘结；肝胆火热上扰，则头晕，口苦口渴；肝胆横逆犯胃，胃失和降，则脘腹胀满，呕恶纳呆；舌质红，舌苔根部黄厚腻，为湿热内蕴、上蒸之征；脉弦滑数，示肝胆有热。

Syndrome analysis: internal accumulation of dampness-heat in the middle energizer fumigates the liver and gallbladder and makes the bile overflow, thus results in yellowed skin and sclera. Heat is a yang pathogen and causes the body as bright yellow as orange. Heat consuming body fluid and excess of yang-ming fu-organ causes fever, thirst, scanty and dark urine and constipation. Fire of the liver and gallbladder goes upward, leading to dizziness, bitter taste in the mouth and thirst. Liver and gallbladder transversely attacking stomach makes it fail to descend, thus leading to abdominal fullness and distention, nausea, vomiting and anorexia. Red tongue with yellow, thick and greasy fur at its root are the signs of internal accumulation and upward fumigation of dampness-heat. Wiry, slippery and rapid pulse shows heat in the liver and gallbladder.

2011 年 8 月 18 日二诊：皮肤及巩膜黄染变浅，脘腹痞满、呕恶不食物症状减轻，大便隔日一行，小便黄赤，舌淡红，苔根部黄腻（图 3.2.2.9b），脉弦滑。前方减生大黄，加土茯苓 15g、金钱草 30g，继服 7 剂，身、面黄染尽退，二便调，纳食增加，余症悉除。肝功能示：谷丙转氨酶 32U/L, 谷草转氨酶 29U/L，碱性磷酸酶 81U/L，谷氨酸转移酶 30U/L，直接胆红素 2.7μmol/L，间接胆红素 6.3μmol/L。

Second visit on August 18, 2011: yellowed skin and sclera were decreased and symptoms of abdominal distention and fullness, nausea, vomiting and anorexia were relieved. The patient had once defecation every other day, brown urine, light red tongue with yellow greasy fur at its root (Fig.3.2.2.9b), and wiry slippery pulse. Seven doses of the previous prescription were used for treatment, with the reduction of shengdahuang but with the addition of tufuling 15g and jinqiancao 30g. After medication, the yellowed skin and sclera disappeared, urine and stool became normal, appetite got improved and other abnormal symptoms all were removed. Liver function: ALT 32U/L, AST 29U/L, ALP 81U/L, GGT 30U/L, DBIL 2.7μmol/L, IBIL 6.3μmol/L.

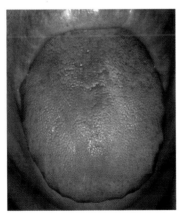 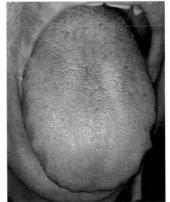

图 3.2.2.9a　　　　　　　　　图 3.2.2.9b
Fig.3.2.2.9a　　　　　　　　Fig.3.2.2.9b

（十）头痛 – 寒滞肝经证

2.10　Headache: syndrome of cold stagnating in the liver meridian

患者刘某，女，40 岁，头痛 10 余年加重 3 天，于 2013 年 11 月 10 日就诊。

Patient Liu, female, 40 years old, had been suffering from headache for more than 10 years and the symptom aggravated 3 days ago. Then she visited the doctor on August 21, 2013.

患者自诉头痛有 10 余年，每于冬令发作，时作时止，夜间尤甚，且颠顶痛甚，痛甚时彻夜不寐，有时有呕吐痰涎。近日头痛症状加重，夜间痛甚，有胃脘嘈杂伴呕吐清水痰涎。患者纳食可，大小便可，无腹痛、腹胀，无吐酸，舌质淡，苔白腻（图 3.2.2.10a），脉象沉弦，重按无力。

The patient had a headache for more than 10 years that often attacked intermittently in winter every year, especially at night. The calvaria headache was severer, which kept her awake all night and sometimes vomited saliva and sputum. Recently, it became much more serious especially at night, accompanied with gastric discomfort and vomiting of clear saliva and sputum. The patient had normal appetite, normal urine and stool, no abdominal pain or distention, no acid regurgitation, pale tongue with white greasy fur (Fig.3.2.2.10a), and deep, wiry pulse that was weak when pressed forcefully.

西医诊断：头痛。

Western medicine diagnosis: headache.

中医诊断：头痛。

TCM diagnosis: headache.

辨证：寒滞肝经证。

Syndrome differentiation: cold stagnation in the liver meridian.

治疗：温阳通降。

Treatment: warming yang and descending turbid.

处方：吴茱萸汤合玉真丸加减：吴茱萸 5g，炒党参 12g，姜半夏 10g，茯苓 15g，川芎 5g，煅钟乳石 15g，制硫黄 1g，马牙硝 1g，生姜 3 片，大枣 5 枚。7 剂，日 1 剂，水煎服。

Prescription: modified *Wuzhuyu* Decoction together with *Yuzhen* Pill.

Wuzhuyu 5g, chaodangshen 12g, jiangbanxia 10g, fuling 15g, chuanxiong 5g, duanzhongrushi 15g, zhiliuhuang 15g, mayaxiao 1g, shengjiang 3 pieces, dazao 5 pieces. 7 doses and one dose a day, decoction.

证候分析：足厥阴肝经上行至颠顶，肝寒犯胃，浊阴之气上逆而至颠顶，出现颠顶痛；肝寒犯胃，胃阳不布产生涎沫随浊气上逆而吐出，见胃脘嘈杂伴呕吐清水痰涎；舌质淡，苔白腻为寒湿内盛之象；脉象沉弦，重按无力为寒阻肝经之征。

Syndrome analysis: since the liver meridian of Foot-Jueyin ascends to the calvaria, liver-cold attacking the stomach and turbid yin ascending to the calvaria cause calvaria headache; liver-cold attacking the stomach and stomach-yang failing to spread cause adverse-rising of turbid qi and gastric discomfort and vomiting of clear saliva and sputum; pale tongue with white greasy fur is the typical manifestation of internal exuberance of cold-dampness; deep wiry and weak pulse indicates cold obstruction of liver meridian.

2013 年 11 月 17 日二诊：头痛明显减轻，胃脘嘈杂缓解，舌淡红，苔白稍腻（图 3.2.2.10b），诊脉濡软而细。原方加生石决明 15g、熟附子 6g，继服 7 剂。随访 1 年，未再头痛。

Second visit on November 17, 2013: the headache was obviously alleviated, and the gastric discomfort was also alleviated. The tongue was light red with white and slightly greasy fur (Fig.3.2.2.10b), and the pulse was soggy, soft and thready. Seven doses of the previous prescription were used for treatment, with the addition of shengshijueming 15g and shufuzi 6g. There was no recurrence of headache according to the feedback one year later.

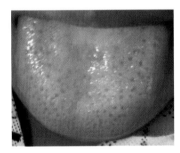 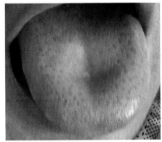

图 3.2.2.10a
Fig.3.2.2.10a

图 3.2.2.10b
Fig.3.2.2.10b

（十一）转筋 – 肝络失养证

2.11 Twitch: symptom of insufficient nourishment of liver collateral

患者田某，男，66 岁，左侧小腿夜间抽搐 2 个月，于 2016 年 4 月 12 日就诊。

Patient Tian, male, 66 years old, had been suffering from spasm in the left leg at night for 2 months, and he visited the doctor on April 12, 2016.

刻诊：形体消瘦，精神可，小腿部夜间抽搐，以左侧小腿为主，右侧小腿偶尔抽搐，抽搐时小腿部肌肉僵硬，疼痛较甚，持续 3 ～ 5 分钟不等，无畏寒、怕冷，纳差，无口干、口苦，无恶心、呕吐，夜寐差，无腰膝酸软、易怒，小便平，大便偏干，舌质红偏瘦，苔薄白（图 3.2.2.11a），脉沉细。

Present symptoms: emaciation, normal spirit, spasm in the left leg at night (and the right leg occasionally had spasm). The spasm was often serious and continued for 3-5 minutes with the calf muscles being stiff. The patient had no aversion to cold, poor appetite, no thirst and bitter taste in the mouth, no nausea and vomiting, poor sleep, no soreness and weakness of waist and knees, no irritability, normal urine and slightly dry stool, red and slightly thin tongue with white thin fur (Fig.3.2.2.11a), and deep thready pulse.

西医诊断：腓肠肌痉挛。

Western medicine diagnosis: gastrocnemius spasm.

中医诊断：转筋。

TCM diagnosis: spasm.

辨证：肝血不足，筋脉失养证。

Syndrome differentiation: liver blood insufficiency, insufficient nourishment of tendons and vessels.

治疗：养血柔肝，舒筋止痛。

Treatment: nourishing blood and emolliating liver, relaxing sinew and relieving pain.

处方：四君子汤合六味地黄汤加减：党参 15g，白芍 20g，当归 12g，川芎 10g，骨碎补 15g，熟地黄 10g，怀牛膝 20g，千年健 15g，鸡血藤 15g，白术 15g，茯苓 15g，夜交藤 30g，谷芽 15g，麦芽 15g，炙甘草 5g。7 剂，日 1 剂，水煎服。

Prescription: modified *Sijunzi* Decoction together with *Liuwei Dihuang* Decoction.

Dangshen 15g, baishao 20g, danggui 12g, chuanxiong 10g, gusuibu 15g, shudihuang 10g, huainiuxi 20g, qiannianjian 15g, jixueteng 15g, baizhu 15g, fuling 15g, yejiaoteng 30g, guya 15g, maiya 15g, zhigancao 5g.

Seven doses and one dose a day, decoction.

证候分析：平素脾胃虚弱，纳食差，气血生化不足，日久致肝血不足；肝藏血，主筋，肝血不足，筋脉失养，则抽搐；肝血不足，血不养心，则失眠；肝阴血不足，肝阳偏亢，则性情急躁易怒；舌质红偏瘦，为阴虚不足，舌体失养所致；脉沉细，为肝血不足、脉道不充之征象。

Syndrome analysis: long-term deficiency of spleen and stomach, poor appetite and insufficient generation and transformation of qi and blood leads to deficiency of liver-blood. And the liver stores blood and governs tendons. Therefore, deficiency of liver-blood and insufficient nourishment of tendons and vessels bring about spasm. Deficiency of liver-blood and blood failing to nourish the heart cause insomnia. Deficiency of liver-blood and hyperactivity of liver yang leads to irritability. Red and slightly thin tongue is the result of yin deficiency and insufficient nourishment of the tongue. Deep and thready pulse is the typical manifestation of deficiency of liver-blood and malnutrition of the vessels.

2016 年 4 月 19 日二诊：患者自诉服上药第 3 剂后，小腿未再抽搐，纳食一般，夜寐差，舌淡红，苔薄白（图 3.2.2.11b），余无异常。守前方加合欢花 20g、山楂 10g，继服 5 剂。

Second visit on April 19, 2016: there was no leg spasm after taking 3 doses of the prescription. And the patient had normal appetite, poor sleep, pale red tongue with thin white fur (Fig.3.2.2.11b), and no other abnormal symptoms. Five doses of the previous prescription were used for treatment, with the addition of hehuanhua 20g and shanzha 10g.

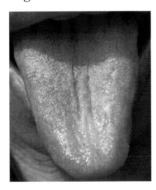 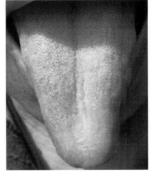

图 3.2.2.11a　　　　　　　　图 3.2.2.11b
Fig.3.2.2.11a　　　　　　　Fig.3.2.2.11b

（十二）震颤 – 肝肾阴虚证

2.12　Tremor: syndrome of yin deficiency of liver and kidney

患者林某，女，78 岁，头摇、双上肢抖动 3 年加重 3 个月，于 2016 年 6 月 11

日就诊。

Patient Lin, female, 78 years old, had been suffering from head shaking and upper limb tremor for 3 years and the symptoms aggravated three months ago. Then she visited the doctor on June 6, 2016.

患者 3 年前出现不自主头摇、双上肢抖动，日渐加重，于当地医院就诊，诊断为"帕金森病"，间断服药控制。近 3 月来，其症状逐渐加重。刻诊：形体消瘦，神志清楚，语言清晰，头部及双上肢不间断地摇动伴头目眩晕，偶有耳鸣，腰膝酸软，失眠多梦，健忘，无恶心、呕吐，纳可，夜尿多，大便干结，舌质暗红，苔薄稍黄（图3.2.2.12a），脉沉细弦。

Three years ago, the patient presented with involuntary head shaking and upper limb tremor that became severer and severer, so she visited the doctor at the local hospital and was diagnosed as Parkinson disease. The patient took medicine discontinuously to control the disease condition. During the latest 3 months the condition became much more serious, so she came to visit the doctor. Present symptoms: emaciation, conscious mind, clear speech, continuous head shaking and upper limb tremor, accompanied with dizziness, occasional tinnitus, soreness and weakness of waist and knees, insomnia and dreaminess, amnesia, no nausea and vomiting, normal appetite, frequent urination at night, dry stool, dark red tongue with thin and slightly yellow fur (Fig.3.2.2.12a), and deep, thready and wiry pulse.

西医诊断：帕金森病。

Western medicine diagnosis: Parkinson disease.

中医诊断：震颤。

TCM diagnosis: tremor.

辨证：肝肾阴亏，筋脉失养证。

Syndrome differentiation: yin deficiency of liver and kidney, insufficient nourishment of tendons and vessels.

治疗：滋补肝肾，养阴柔筋。

Treatment: nourishing liver and kidney, nourishing yin and emolliating tendons.

处方：一贯煎加减：玄参 30g，生地黄 15g，山药 15g，丹参 15g，当归 10g，白芍 10g，山茱萸 10g，茯苓 15g，杜仲 15g，生龟甲 30g（先煎），生鳖甲 30g（先煎），钩藤 15g，肉苁蓉 15g，火麻仁 15g。7 剂，日 1 剂，水煎服。

Prescription: modified *Yiguan* Decoction.

Xuanshen 30g, shengdihuang 15g, shanyao 15g, danshen 15g, danggui 10g, baishao 10g, shanzhuyu 10g, fuling 15g, duzhong 15g, shengguijia 30g (decocted first), shengbiejia 30g (decocted first), gouteng 15g, roucongrong 15g, huomaren 15g.

Seven doses and one dose a day, decoction.

证候分析：患者年老体衰，正气亏虚，肝肾精血不足，肝不藏血，肾不藏精，则筋脉髓海失养，而见头摇、肢颤等虚风内动之象；肝之阴血不足，阴不制阳，风阳上扰，则头晕目眩；心神不宁而失眠多梦；肾精不足，腰府失养，则腰膝酸软；肾精不足，脑海不充，则脑转耳鸣；肾司二便，肾阴不足，肠道失濡，则大便干结；阴血亏虚，血行迟缓，则致瘀，故舌质暗红；少苔、脉沉细弦，均为阴血不足之象。

Syndrome analysis: the patient's multiple-pathogenesis of old age, weak constitution, healthy qi deficiency, and essence and blood insufficiency of the liver and kidney as well as the liver failing to store blood and the kidney failing to store essence causes improper nourishment of the tendons, vessels and marrow, so head shaking and upper limb tremor happen which are the manifestations of internal stirring of deficient wind; deficiency of liver-blood and yin failing to control yang cause wind-yang upward disturbs the clear orifice, so dizziness, and disquieted heart spirit with insomnia and dreaminess. Deficiency of kidney essence with improper nourishment of the waist leads to soreness and weakness of waist and knees. Deficiency of kidney essence with improper nourishment of the brain causes vertigo and tinnitus. Deficiency of kidney yin with insufficient moistening of the intestines triggers dry stool. Deficiency of yin-blood and slow blood circulation cause blood stasis, so the tongue is dark red. The tongue with little fur, and the deep, thready and wiry pulse，are the manifestations of deficiency of blood and yin.

2016 年 6 月 18 日二诊：患者仍有头摇肢颤，但头目眩晕症状减轻，肢体有力，夜寐差，大便正常，夜尿多，舌质暗，苔薄白（图 3.2.2.12b），脉沉细。原方加夜交藤 30g、合欢皮 20g、益智仁 20g，14 剂，继续调理。

Second visit on June 18, 2016: the patient still had head shaking and upper limb tremor while dizziness was relieved. The patient felt stronger limbs, poor sleep, normal stool, frequent urination at night, dark tongue with thin white fur (Fig.3.2.2.12b), and deep thready pulse. 14 doses of the previous prescription were used for treatment, with the addition of yejiaoteng 30g, hehuanpi 20g and yizhiren 20g.

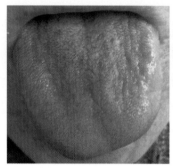 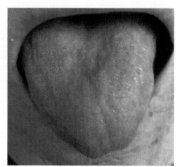

图 3.2.2.12a   图 3.2.2.12b

Fig.3.2.2.12a   Fig.3.2.2.12b

三、脾胃系病证

3. Spleen and stomach disease syndrome

（一）胃痛 – 心脾两虚证

3.1 Stomachache: syndrome of deficiency of both heart and spleen

患者李某，女，39 岁，胃痛胃胀 3 年加重 1 月，于 2016 年 7 月 20 日就诊。

Patient Li, female, 39 years old, had been suffering from pain and distention in stomach for 3 years. The symptoms got aggravated one month ago, so she came to visit the doctor on July 20, 2016.

患者患胃痛、胃胀不适 3 年，间断服中西药物治疗，但症状易于反复，近 1 月来胃痛症状加重而就诊。刻诊：精神差，焦虑貌，自诉胃脘隐痛作胀，食后稍舒，偶有恶心、反酸，口不渴，失眠，多梦易醒，烦躁易怒，二便平，舌淡紫胖大有齿痕，苔黄白相间（图 3.2.3.1a），脉缓弱。胃镜检查示：非萎缩性胃炎伴糜烂。

The patient had been suffering from stomach pain and distention for 3 years, during which she took traditional Chinese and Western medicine on and off, but the symptoms occurred repeatedly. She visited the doctor due to the increasing stomachache about one month ago. Present symptoms: listlessness, anxiety, epigastric dull pain and distention which can be relieved after eating, nausea and acid regurgitation (sometimes), no thirst, insomnia, dreaminess and easy wake-up, dysphoria, irritability, and normal urine and stool, pale purple, enlarged and teeth-marked tongue with yellow white fur (Fig.3.2.3.1a), and moderate weak pulse. Gastroscopy: non-atrophic gastritis with erosion.

西医诊断：非萎缩性胃炎伴糜烂。

Western medicine diagnosis: non-atrophic gastritis with erosion.

中医诊断：胃痛。

TCM diagnosis: stomachache.

辨证：心脾两虚伴肝胃不和证。

Syndrome differentiation: heart-spleen deficiency and liver-stomach disharmony.

治疗：健脾养心，和胃止痛。

Treatment: invigorating spleen and nourishing stomach, harmonizing stomach and relieving pain.

处方：归脾汤加减：党参 15g，黄芪 15g，白术 15g，茯苓 15g，陈皮 6g，香附 6g，桂枝 6g，白芍 10g，远志 10g，旋覆花 15g（包煎），炒酸枣仁 20g，龙眼肉 15g，生姜 3 片，大枣 5 枚。7 剂，日 1 剂，水煎服。

Prescription: modified *Guipi* Decoction.

Dangshen 15g, huangqi 15g, baizhu 15g, fuling 15g, chenpi 6g, xiangfu 6g, guizhi 6g, baishao 10g, yuanzhi 10g, xuanfuhua 15g (wrap-boiling), chaosuanzaoren 20g, longyanrou 15g, shengjiang 3 pieces, dazao 5 pieces.

Seven doses and one dose a day, decoction.

证候分析：脾气亏虚，生化气血不足，血不养心致心血虚而见失眠；脾虚不运，胃降失职，则见恶心、反酸；脾胃气滞而见胃脘胀痛不舒；食后气机得助，则疼痛减轻；肝气不舒，则烦躁易怒；肝气犯胃，加重胃脘胀痛；舌质淡紫，舌体胖大伴齿痕，苔黄白相间，为脾虚不运，水湿内停之象；脉缓弱，为正虚不足之征。

Syndrome analysis: spleen qi deficiency fails to produce sufficient qi and blood, and causes insufficient nourishment of the heart, so insomnia occurs. Stomach qi failing to descend causes nausea and acid regurgitation. Spleen-stomach qi stagnation causes epigastric distending pain which can get relieved when food taking supports qi movement. Constraining of liver qi causes dysphoria and irritability. Liver qi invading stomach aggravates distending pain. Pale purple, enlarged and teeth-marked tongue with yellow white fur indicate that spleen deficiency fails to transport food and water, thus leading to water-dampness retention. Moderate and weak pulse is the manifestation of healthy qi deficiency.

2016 年 7 月 27 日二诊：胃脘部疼痛减轻，偶有反酸，无恶心，夜寐 5 小时左右，舌淡，苔白（图 3.2.3.1b），脉弱。原方加海螵蛸 20g、瓦楞子 15g、夜交藤 30g，7 剂，继续治疗。

Second visit on July 27, 2016: the patient had alleviated epigastric pain, occasionally acid regurgitation, no nausea, sleep time about 5 hours every day, pale tongue with white fur (Fig.3.2.3.1b), and weak pulse.

Seven doses of the previous prescription were used for treatment with the addition of haipiaoxiao 20g, walengzi 15g, and yejiaoteng 30g.

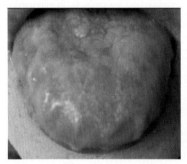 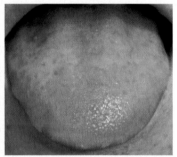

图 3.2.3.1a　　　　　　　　　图 3.2.3.1b
Fig.3.2.3.1a　　　　　　　　　Fig.3.2.3.1b

（二）胃痛 – 肝气犯胃证

3.2　Stomachache: syndrome of liver qi invading stomach

患者章某，女，58 岁，上腹间断隐痛 20 年加重 1 月，于 2016 年 11 月 10 日就诊。

Patient Zhang, female, 58 years old, had been suffering from upper abdominal intermittent dull pain for 20 years. The symptom got aggravated one month ago, so she came to visit the doctor on January 10, 2016.

患者上腹胃脘部间断隐痛 20 年，胃镜检查示胃多发性息肉，服中西药物治疗，但症状时有反复。近 1 月来，患者上腹隐痛、反酸症状加重遂来就诊。刻诊：精神差，焦虑貌，自诉上腹隐痛，伴嘈杂、反酸、烧心，空腹时加重，进食后稍减，纳食尚可，夜寐不安、难入睡，平素性情暴躁，易于烦躁、焦虑，二便平，舌质淡暗，苔白腻而干（图 3.2.3.2a），脉沉弦。胃镜检查示：胃多发性息肉，胃底黏膜隆起，非萎缩性胃炎。活检示：胃底腺息肉。

The patient had been suffering from intermittent dull pain in the epigastric part for 20 years. The endoscopy showed multiple gastric polyps. She took Chinese and Western medicine drugs, but the symptom was repeated. In recent a month, the symptoms of dull pain and acid regurgitation became severe, so she came to visit the doctor. Present symptoms: listlessness, anxiety, dull pain in the upper abdomen accompanied by epigastric upset, acid regurgitation and heartburn (which could get aggravated before meals and slightly relieved after meals), normal appetite, poor sleep, difficulty in falling asleep, irritability, dysphoria, normal urine and stool, light dark tongue with white greasy and dry fur (Fig.3.2.3.2a), and deep wiry pulse. Gastroscopy: multiple gastric polyps, gastric submucosal humus, and non-atrophic gastritis. Biopsy: gastric fundus polyp.

西医诊断：胃多发性息肉。

Western medicine diagnosis: multiple polyps of stomach.

中医诊断：胃痛；郁证。

TCM diagnosis: stomachache; depression syndrome.

辨证：肝气郁结，横逆犯胃证。

Syndrome differentiation: liver qi depression transversely invading stomach.

治疗：疏肝和胃，理气止痛。

Treatment: soothing liver and harmonizing stomach, regulating qi and relieving pain.

处方：柴胡疏肝散加减：党参 15g，白术 15g，茯苓 15g，半夏 10g，陈皮 8g，乌贼骨 15g，柴胡 10g，白芍 15g，甘草 6g，枳壳 10g，川楝子 10g，延胡索 15g。7 剂，日 1 剂，水煎服。

Prescription: modified *Chaihu Shugan* Powder.

Dangshen 15g, baizhu 15g, fuling 15g, banxia 10g, chenpi 8g, wuzeigu 15g, chaihu 10g, baishao 15g, gancao 6g, zhiqiao 10g, chuanlianzi 10g, yanhusuo 15g.

Seven doses and one dose a day, decoction.

证候分析：肝主疏泄，以条达为顺，因情志不遂，肝气郁结，横逆犯胃，胃失和降，则胃脘胀痛，胸脘痞闷；胃气上逆，则上腹隐痛，伴嘈杂、反酸、烧心；肝气郁久，则血行不畅，血脉凝涩，可见舌质暗淡；苔白、脉沉弦，为肝气郁滞之象。

Syndrome analysis: since liver governs free flow of qi and likes stretching, liver qi depression invades stomach due to long emotional frustration; when stomach qi fails to descend, epigastric distending pain and chest stuffiness occur; when stomach qi flows upwards, there is dull pain in the upper abdomen, accompanied by epigastric upset, acid regurgitation and heartburn; when liver qi depression lasts, blood cannot circulate smoothly and even stagnates, and light dark tongue can be seen; white fur and deep wiry pulse indicate liver qi depression and obstruction.

2016 年 11 月 17 日二诊：胃脘疼痛明显减轻，偶有反酸、烧心，夜寐 5 ～ 6 小时，舌质淡红，苔薄白（图 3.2.3.2b），脉弦。原方加黄连 6g、吴茱萸 1g、茯神 20g，7 剂，继续治疗。

Second visit on November 17, 2016: the patient had alleviated gastric pain, occasionally acid regurgitation and burning sensation, sleep time about five or six hours every day, pale red tongue with thin and white fur (Fig.3.2.3.2b), and wiry pulse.

Seven doses of the previous prescription were used for treatment with the addition of huanglian 6g, wuzhuyu 1g, and fushen 20g.

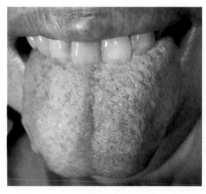 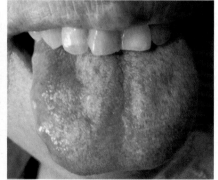

图 3.2.3.2a　　　　　　　　　图 3.2.3.2b
Fig.3.2.3.2a　　　　　　　　Fig.3.2.3.2b

（三）胃痛 – 湿热内蕴证

3.3　Stomachache: syndrome of internal accumulation of dampness-heat

患者盛某，女，33 岁，上腹部灼痛 2 月余，于 2017 年 5 月 6 日就诊。

Patient Sheng, female, 33 years old, had been suffering from upper abdominal burning pain for more than 2 months, then she came to visit the doctor on May 6, 2017.

患者 2 个月前不明原因出现上腹部灼痛，行胃镜检查示轻度胃溃疡，自行服药（具体不详）后症状略有好转，为求进一治疗而就诊。刻诊：自诉上腹部灼痛，食凉减轻，平素喜食辛辣食物，后咽喉部灼痛，偶感反酸，呕吐，烧心，纳可，寐安，口干喜冷饮，小便平，大便 3 ~ 4 日一行，质偏干，舌质红，苔薄黄（图 3.2.3.3a），脉滑数，左脉关部弦细，右脉关部沉实。

The patient felt an unknown burning pain in the upper abdomen two months ago. Gastroscopy indicated mild gastric ulcer. She took medication at home by herself and the symptoms were relieved slightly. In order to get a further treatment, she went to see the doctor. Present symptoms: burning pain in the upper abdomen which could be relieved after eating cold food, preference for spicy food, burning pain in the posterior part of throat, occasionally acid regurgitation and vomiting, heartburn, normal appetite and sleep, dry mouth and desire to take cold drink, normal urine, slightly dry stool with defecation 3-4 times a day, red tongue with thin yellow fur (Fig.3.2.3.3a), and slippery rapid pulse with left guan wiry and thready, and right guan deep and replete.

西医诊断：胃溃疡。

Western medicine diagnosis: gastric ulcer.

中医诊断：胃痛。

TCM diagnosis: stomachache.

辨证：湿热中阻，胃气不降证。

Syndrome differentiation: dampness-heat obstruction in the middle, stomach qi failing to descend.

治疗：清热化湿，和胃降逆。

Treatment: clearing heat and resolving dampness, harmonizing stomach and descending adverse qi.

处方：黄连温胆汤加减：太子参 15g，黄连 10g，厚朴 10g，枳壳 10g，白术 15g，姜半夏 10g，竹茹 15g，陈皮 8g，薏苡仁 20g，山药 20g，郁金 12g，延胡索 15g，肉苁蓉 15g，甘草 6g。7 剂，日 1 剂，水煎服。

Prescription: modified *Huanglian Wendan* Decoction.

Taizishen 15g, huanglian 10g, houpo 10g, zhiqiao 10g, baizhu 15g, jiangbanxia 10g, zhuru 15g, chenpi 8g, yiyiren 20g, shanyao 20g, yujin 12g, yanhusuo 15g, roucongrong 15g, gancao 6g.

Seven doses and one dose a day, decoction.

证候分析：平素过食辛辣，湿热内蕴，则烧心，上腹部灼痛；胃气通降受阻，湿热之邪随胃气上逆，则后咽喉部灼痛，偶感反酸，呕吐；湿热蕴脾，上蒸于口，故口干喜冷饮；湿热下注，阻碍气机，大肠传导失司，故大便秘结；舌质红，苔薄黄，为邪热熏灼于舌之征；脉滑数，为湿热内蕴之象。

Syndrome analysis: overeating spicy food results in dampness-heat internal accumulation, and further leads to heartburn and burning pain in the upper abdomen; when obstructed stomach qi fails to descend, dampness-heat goes up, causing burning pain in the posterior part of the throat, occasional acid regurgitation and vomiting; when dampness-heat accumulation in the spleen rises to steam the mouth, the patient has a dry mouth and prefers cold drink; when dampness-heat pours down to obstruct qi movement and cause dysfunction of intestinal conveyance, constipation emerges; red tongue and thin yellow fur tells that heat pathogen fumigates and scorches the tongue; slippery and rapid pulse indicates internal accumulation of dampness-heat.

2017 年 5 月 13 日二诊：上腹灼痛症状减轻，偶有反酸，无呕吐，口干，二便平，舌淡红，苔薄白（图 3.2.3.3b），脉弦。原方加海螵蛸 15g、浙贝母 10g、麦冬 10g，7 剂，继续治疗。

Second visit on May 13,2017: the patient had relieved burning pain in the upper abdomen, occasional acid regurgitation, no vomiting, dry mouth, normal urine and stool, pale tongue with thin and white fur (Fig.3.2.3.3b), and wiry pulse. Seven doses of the previous prescription were used for treatment with the addition of haipiaoxiao 15g, zhebeimu 10g, and maidong 10g.

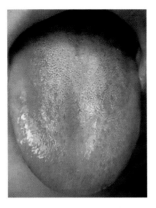
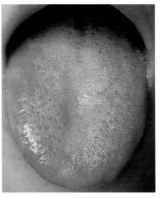

图 3.2.3.3a
Fig.3.2.3.3a

图 3.2.3.3b
Fig.3.2.3.3b

（四）胃痞 – 肝郁脾虚证

3.4 Stomach stuffiness: syndrome of liver depression and spleen deficiency

患者林某，女，57 岁，胃脘嘈杂、反酸 10 余年加重 1 月，于 2017 年 4 月 20 日就诊。

Patient Lin, female, 57 years old, had been suffering from epigastric upset and acid regurgitation for 10 years with these symptoms aggravated one month ago, so she came to visit the doctor on January 20, 2017.

患者胃病 10 多年，曾中西药物治疗（具体用药不详），但症状反复发作。近 1 月来患者因情志不和而致胃脘嘈杂、反酸症状加重，遂来就诊。刻诊：精神差，神疲乏力，自诉进食后自觉腹中有气向上冲逆，泛酸，纳可，易于烦躁，夜寐不安，多梦易醒，小便平，大便不规律，日 2 ～ 3 次，干结不调，舌暗淡，苔白腻（图 3.2.3.4a），脉弦。胃镜检查示：非萎缩性胃炎伴糜烂。腹部 B 超示：左肾结石。咽喉镜示：慢性咽炎。

The patient had been suffering from gastrosis for more than 10 years, and treated with Chinese and Western medicine (specific medication was unknown), but the symptoms still occurred repeatedly. In recent one month, the symptom of epigastric upset and acid regurgitation became aggravated due to emotional factors. And then she came to see the doctor. Present symptoms: listlessness, lacking of strength, qi rushing upwards after eating, acid regurgitation, normal appetite, dysphoria, poor sleep, dreaminess, easy wake-up, normal urine, irregular defecation with dry or loose stool 2-3 times a day, light dark tongue with white greasy fur (Fig.3.2.3.4a), and wiry pulse. Gastroscopy: non-atrophic gastritis with erosion. Abdominal B: left kidney stone. Laryngeal mirror: chronic pharyngitis.

西医诊断：非萎缩性胃炎伴糜烂；焦虑症。

Western medicine diagnosis: non-atrophic gastritis with erosion; anxiety disorders.

中医诊断：胃痞。

TCM diagnosis: stomach stuffiness.

辨证：肝郁脾虚证。

Syndrome differentiation: liver depression and spleen deficiency.

治疗：疏肝健脾，行气和胃。

Treatment: soothing liver and invigorating spleen, moving qi and harmonizing stomach.

处方：柴胡疏肝散加减：党参 15g，炒白术 15g，桑螵蛸 15g，茯苓 15g，柴胡 6g，枳壳 10g，厚朴 10g，白芍 20g，当归 10g，牡丹皮 9g，谷麦 10g，麦芽 10g，泽泻 10g。7 剂，日 1 剂，水煎服。

Prescription: modified *Chaihu Shugan* Powder.

Dangshen 15g, chaobaizhu 15g, sangpiaoxiao 15g, fuling 15g, chaihu 6g, zhiqiao 10g, houpo 10g, baishao 20g, danggui 10g, mudanpi 9g, guya 10g, maiya 10g, zexie 10g.

Seven doses and one dose a day, decoction.

证候分析：肝气郁结，横逆犯脾，脾气不运，影响于胃，出现胃脘不适，食后气机受阻，则腹胀更甚；肝郁日久化火，内扰胃府，胃气上逆，出现胃脘嘈杂、反酸；肝郁脾虚，则见大便干稀不调；舌暗淡，苔白腻，脉弦，为肝郁脾虚之征。

Syndrome analysis: when liver qi depression transversely invades the spleen, the spleen qi failing to transport causes stomach discomfort (abdominal distention becomes severer after eating since food taking blocks qi movement); when persistent liver qi depression transforms into fire which harasses the stomach, stomach qi rises reversely, and gastric upset and acid regurgitation happen; liver depression and spleen deficiency lead to irregular defecation with dry or loose stool; light dark tongue with white greasy fur and wiry pulse serve as the manifestations of liver depression and spleen deficiency.

2017 年 4 月 27 日二诊：患者精神较前好转，胃脘嘈杂、反酸症状减轻，腹中气上逆不减，夜寐差，纳食可，大便日 1 ~ 2 次，舌淡红，苔白（图 3.2.3.4b），脉弦。原方加代赭石 20g、紫苏子 10g、夜交藤 30g、茯神 20g，7 剂。

Second visit on April 27, 2017: the patient had improved spirit, relieved gastric upset and acid regurgitation, stomach qi ascending counterflow, poor sleep, normal appetite, defecation once or twice a day, light red tongue with white fur (Fig.3.2.3.4b), and wiry pulse.

Seven doses of the previous prescription were used for consolidation with the addition of daizheshi 20g, zisuzi 10g, yejiaoteng 30g, and fushen 20g.

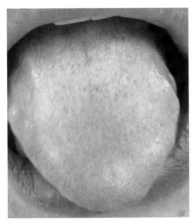 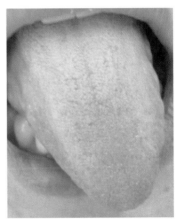

图 3.2.3.4a
Fig.3.2.3.4a

图 3.2.3.4b
Fig.3.2.3.4b

（五）胃痞－脾虚湿困证

3.5 Stomach stuffiness: syndrome of spleen deficiency and dampness encumbering

患者吴某，男，62 岁，胃病多年加重 10 天，于 2017 年 4 月 13 日就诊。

Patient Wu, male, 62 years old, had been suffering from stomach illness for many years. It became aggravated 10 days ago, and thus he came to visit the doctor on April 13, 2017.

患者胃病多年，曾行胃镜检查示：非萎缩性胃炎伴糜烂，十二指肠球炎。近 10 天来因患者饮食不慎出现胃脘部胀闷不适而就诊。刻诊：精神可，自诉上腹胀满痞闷伴嘈杂，食后痞满更甚，纳食差，周身乏力，无恶心、呕吐，无反酸、嗳气，寐可，二便平，舌质淡胖有齿痕、苔白腻（图 3.2.3.5a），脉濡缓。

The patient had been suffering from stomach illness for many years. The gastroscopy indicated non-atrophic gastritis with erosion, and duodenitis. The patient had been suffering from epigastric fullness because of his improper diet for 10 days, therefore he came to see the doctor. Present symptoms: normal mental state, stuffiness and fullness in the upper abdomen with noise, severer stuffiness and fullness after eating, poor appetite, general fatigue, no nausea and vomiting, no acid regurgitation and belching, normal sleep, normal urine and stool, pale enlarged and teeth-marked tongue with white greasy fur (Fig.3.2.3.5a), and soggy moderate pulse.

西医诊断：非萎缩性胃炎伴糜烂；十二指肠球炎。

Western medicine diagnosis: non-atrophic gastritis with erosion, duodenitis.

中医诊断：胃痞。

TCM diagnosis: stomach stuffiness.

辨证：脾虚湿困，中焦不运证。

Syndrome differentiation: spleen deficiency with dampness encumbering, dysfunction of the middle energizer in transportation.

治疗：健脾利湿，消痞除满。

Treatment: invigorating spleen and draining dampness, dispersing abdominal stuffiness and removing fullness.

处方：补中益气汤加减：黄芪 25g，党参 6g，炒白术 10g，升麻 6g，香橼 10g，陈皮 6g，炙甘草 10g，茯苓 15g，泽泻 10g，白芍 12g，砂仁 6g，鸡内金 10g，丹参 12g，清半夏 6g，生姜 6g，大枣 5 枚。7 剂，日 1 剂，水煎服。

Prescription: modified *Buzhong Yiqi* Decoction.

Huangqi 25g, dangshen 6g, chaobaizhu 10g, shengma 6g, xiangyuan 10g, chenpi 6g, zhigancao 10g, fuling 15g, zexie 10g, baishao 12g, sharen 6g, jineijin 10g, danshen 12g, qingbanxia 6g, shengjiang 6g, dazao 5 pieces.

Seven doses and one dose a day, decoction.

证候分析：脾虚不运，影响及胃，脾气不升，胃气不降，停滞中焦，而见胃脘痞闷不适，兼之脾虚运化不足，湿邪阻滞，则痞闷更甚，食后气机阻滞更甚，则胀闷更甚；脾虚不运，四末失养，兼之湿邪所困，则周身乏力；舌质暗淡胖有齿痕，苔白腻，脉濡缓，为脾虚湿困之明证。

Syndrome analysis: spleen deficiency fails to transport, and stomach is thereby affected; when spleen qi fails to ascend and stomach qi fails to descend, the middle energizer is obstructed, so epigastric stuffiness emerges. Spleen deficiency with dysfunction in transportation and transformation causes dampness obstruction, which aggravates the epigastric stuffiness. Qi movement obstruction getting more severe after taking food explains severer stuffiness and fullness after eating. Spleen deficiency with dysfunction in transportation and dampness encumbering the middle causes general fatigue. Light, dark, enlarged and teeth-marked tongue with white greasy fur and soggy moderate pulse indicate spleen deficiency with dampness encumbering.

2017 年 4 月 20 日二诊：患者诉胃脘痞闷不适症状减轻，纳食好转，寐可，二便正常，舌淡胖，苔白（图 3.2.3.5b），脉缓。原方加厚朴 10g、枳壳 10g、紫苏梗 6g，巩固治疗。

Second visit on April 20, 2017: the patient had relieved epigastric stuffiness, better appetite, normal sleep, normal urine and stool, pale and enlarged tongue, white fur (Fig.3.2.3.5b), and moderate pulse. The previous prescription was used for consolidation with the addition of houpo 10g, zhiqiao 10g, and zisugeng 6g.

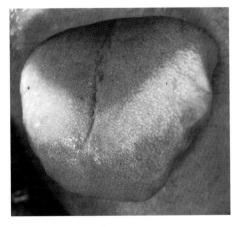

图 3.2.3.5a
Fig.3.2.3.5a

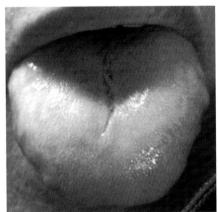

图 3.2.3.5b
Fig.3.2.3.5b

（六）胃痞 – 脾气亏虚证

3.6　Stomach stuffiness: syndrome of depleting spleen qi

患者吴某，男，42 岁，腹部胀闷 5 年加重 1 月，于 2017 年 4 月 5 日就诊。

Patient Wu, male, 42 years old, had been suffering from abdominal distension and stuffiness for 5 years. It became aggravated one month ago, and thus he came to visit the doctor on January 5, 2017.

患者腹部胀闷 5 年，未系统治疗。近 1 月来患者感觉上腹胀闷较前加重，遂来就诊。刻诊：精神差，易疲劳，易汗出，纳差，常感腹胀闷，时轻时重，便后胀痛缓解，寐可，便溏带血，日 2 次，无黏液、脓血，小便平，舌质淡紫，苔白腻（图 3.2.3.6a），脉弱。大便潜血（++）。结肠镜检查示：直肠炎。胃镜检查示：非萎缩性胃炎伴胆汁反流。

The patient had been suffering from abdominal distension and stuffiness for 5 years which had not received systematic treatment. In recent one month, the symptom became aggravated, and therefore he came to see the doctor. Present symptoms: poor mental state, fatigue, easy sweating, poor appetite, abdominal distension and stuffiness (sometimes light, sometimes severe) which can be relieved after defecation, normal sleep, defecation 2 times a day with bloody and loose stool without mucus and pus, normal urine, pale purple tongue with white greasy fur (Fig.3.2.3.6a), and weak pulse. Fecal occult blood (++). Colonoscopy: proctitis. Gastroscopy: non-atrophic gastritis with bile reflux.

西医诊断：直肠炎；非萎缩性胃炎。

Western medicine diagnosis: straight enteritis; non-atrophic gastritis.

中医诊断：胃痞。

TCM diagnosis: stomach stuffiness.

辨证：脾气虚弱，中焦不运证。

Syndrome differentiation: spleen qi deficiency, dysfunction of the middle energizer in transportation.

治疗：健脾益气，消痞除满。

Treatment: invigorating spleen and replenishing qi, dispersing abdominal stuffiness and removing fullness.

处方：四君子汤加减：党参 15g，白术 15g，茯苓 15g，法半夏 10g，枳壳 10g，厚朴 10g，陈皮 6g，紫苏梗 6g，白及 12g，蒲黄炭 15g，干姜 5g，炙甘草 5g。7 剂，日 1 剂，水煎服。

Prescription: modified *Sijunzi* Decoction.

Dangshen 15g, baizhu 15g, fuling 15g, fabanxia 10g, zhiqiao 10g, houpo 10g, chenpi 6g, sugeng 6g, baiji 12g, puhuangtan 15g, ganjiang 5g, zhigancao 5g.

Seven doses and one dose a day, decoction.

证候分析：脾气虚弱，清阳不升，胃之浊阴不降，中焦气机运行受阻，则脘腹胀闷；脾气虚弱，气血生化不足，脏腑功能衰退，则神疲乏力；气虚固摄失司，故自汗；脾虚失运，水湿下注肠道，故便溏；气虚脉道失固，则便中带血；舌质淡紫，苔白腻，脉弱，为脾气亏虚之象。

Syndrome analysis: spleen qi deficiency, lucid yang failing to ascend and turbid yin failing to descend causes qi movement obstruction in the middle energizer, leading to abdominal distention and stuffiness; spleen qi deficiency and adequate generation and transformation of qi and blood cause declining functions of *zang-fu* organs, thus fatigue and lacking of strength occurs; qi deficiency fails to secure the exterior, so spontaneous sweating is caused; dysfunction of the spleen in transportation triggers water-dampness pouring down into the intestines, so loose stool emerges; vessel passage loses control over the blood due to qi deficiency, so the stool is mixed with blood; light purple tongue with white greasy fur and weak pulse indicate the depleting spleen qi.

2017 年 4 月 12 日二诊：患者脘腹胀满症状减轻，纳食增加，精神可，易汗出，大便色黄，舌质淡红，苔白稍腻（图 3.2.3.6b），脉缓。大便潜血（＋）。原方加浮小麦 30g，继续治疗。

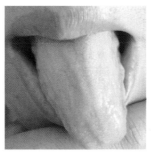 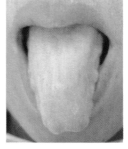

图 3.2.3.6a   图 3.2.3.6b
Fig.3.2.3.6a   Fig.3.2.3.6b

Second visit on April 12, 2017: the patient had relieved abdominal fullness and distention, better appetite, good spirit, easy sweating, yellow stool, pale red tongue with white and slightly greasy fur (Fig.3.2.3.6b), and moderate pulse. Fecal occult blood (+). The previous prescription was used for further treatment with the addition of fuxiaomai 30g.

（七）腹胀 – 肝郁化火证

3.7 Abdominal distension: syndrome of liver depression transforming into fire

患者颜某，女，61 岁，腹胀、嘈杂不适 1 月，于 2016 年 10 月 8 日就诊。

Patient Yan, female, 61 years old, came to visit the doctor on October 8, 2016 due to abdominal distension and epigastric upset for one month.

患者 1 月前因情志不遂致脘腹胀满不适，症状时轻时重，腹胀与精神情志密切相关，为求治疗而就诊。刻诊：精神差，神疲乏力，自诉胸胁胀闷，上腹部胀满呈阵发性，胃脘嘈杂不适，纳差，食后腹胀甚，呃逆，矢气，汗多，易口酸、口臭，易烦躁，睡眠差，大便偏干，小便平，舌质暗红，苔黄腻而干（图 3.2.3.7a），脉弦数。胃镜检查示：非萎缩性胃炎。CT、MIR 检查示：脑动脉硬化缺血。

The patient felt epigastric fullness due to emotional frustration one month ago. The symptom, sometimes relieved and sometimes aggravated, was closely related to emotions. In order to get a further treatment, she went to see the doctor. Present symptoms: poor mental state, lassitude, lacking of strength, chest and hypochondrium distention and oppression, paroxysmal distention and fullness in the upper abdomen, epigastric upset, poor appetite, severer abdominal distention after eating, hiccup, flatus, profuse sweating, sour taste in the mouth, fetid mouth odor, irritability, poor sleep, slightly dry stool, normal urine, dark red tongue with yellow, greasy and dry fur (Fig.3.2.3.7a), and wiry rapid pulse. Gastroscopy: non-atrophic gastritis. Brain CT and MIR: cerebral arteriosclerosis ischemia.

西医诊断：脑动脉供血不足；非萎缩性胃炎。

Western medicine diagnosis: insufficient blood supply of cerebral artery; non atrophic gastritis.

中医诊断：腹胀。

TCM diagnosis: abdominal distension.

辨证：肝郁化火，横逆犯胃证。

Syndrome differentiation: liver depression transforming into fire and transversely invading stomach.

治疗：疏肝解郁清热。

Treatment: soothing liver, relieving depression and clearing heat.

处方：丹栀逍遥散加减：牡丹皮 10g，栀子 10g，柴胡 10g，白术 15g，茯神 20g，白芍 15g，当归 10g，薄荷 6g（后下），蒲公英 15g，陈皮 6g，枳壳 10g，厚朴 10g。7 剂，日 1 剂，水煎服。

Prescription: modified *Danzhi Xiaoyao* Powder.

Mudanpi 10g, zhizi 10g, chaihu 10g, baizhu 15g, fushen 20g, baishao 15g, danggui 10g, bohe 6g (decocted later), pugongying 15g, chenpi 6g, zhiqiao 10g, houpo 10g.

Seven doses and one dose a day, decoction.

证候分析：肝气郁结，情志不畅，则烦躁、易怒；肝郁日久化火犯胃，胃失和降，则脘腹胀满；食后气机阻滞更甚，则胀满更甚；火热熏灼胃腑，浊气上逆，则呃逆、口酸、口臭；肝气郁滞，气机不畅，则胸胁部胀闷；肝郁扰乱心神，则寐差；火热伤阴，则便干；舌质暗红，苔黄腻而干，脉弦数，为肝郁化火之象。

Syndrome analysis: liver qi depression leads to dysphoria and irritability; persistent depression of liver qi transforms into fire and invades the stomach, which causes failure of stomach qi to descend and abdominal distension and fullness; such distention and fullness can get severer when food taking obstructs qi movement; when fire heat fumigates and scorches stomach, turbid qi goes up, causing hiccup, sour taste in the mouth, and fetid mouth odor; when liver qi stagnates and qi movement remains obstructed, chest and hypochondrium distention and oppression emerge; liver qi depression disturbs heart spirit, leading to poor sleep; fire heat damages yin, causing dry stool; liver qi depression transforming into fire is indicated by dark red tongue with yellow, greasy and dry fur and wiry rapid pulse.

2016 年 10 月 15 日二诊：患者精神佳，腹胀减轻，偶有嘈杂、呃逆，纳可，寐差，二便平。舌暗，苔白（图 3.2.3.7b），脉弦。原方加黄连 6g、吴茱萸 1g、煅龙骨 20g、煅牡蛎 20g，7 剂，巩固治疗。

Second visit on October 15, 2016: the patient had good spirit, relieved abdominal distention, occasionally epigastric upset and hiccup, normal appetite, poor sleep, normal urine and stool, dark tongue with white fur (Fig.3.2.3.7b), and wiry pulse.

Seven doses of the previous prescription were used for consolidation with the addition of huanglian 6g, wuzhuyu 1g, duanlonggu 20g, and duanmuli 20g.

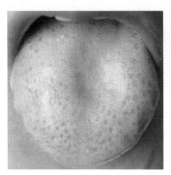 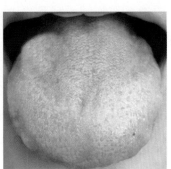

图 3.2.3.7a   图 3.2.3.7b
Fig.3.2.3.7a   Fig.3.2.3.7b

（八）嘈杂 - 脾胃虚弱证

3.8 Epigastric upset: syndrome of deficiency of spleen and stomach

患者乐某，女，46 岁，胃脘部嘈杂不适 1 年余，于 2017 年 5 月 10 日就诊。

Patient Le, female, 46 years old, had been suffering from epigastric upset for more than one year and came to visit the doctor on May 10, 2017.

刻诊：形体消瘦，神疲体倦，自诉空腹时胃脘部嘈杂，食后减轻，伴嗳气、恶心，口淡无味，无呕吐、泛酸、烧心，入睡困难，易醒，小便平，大便不调，舌淡紫伴裂纹，苔黄腻（图 3.2.3.8a），左脉短沉微，右脉沉实，尺部微弱。血常规检查：白细胞计数 4.2×10^9/L，血红蛋白 12g/L，血小板计数 68×10^9/L。胃镜检查示：慢性浅表性胃炎。

Present symptoms: emaciation, fatigue, epigastric upset when stomach is empty and that can be relieved after eating, belching, nausea, bland taste in the mouth, no vomiting, no acid regurgitation and heartburn, difficult sleeping with easy wake-up, normal urine, irregular stool, pale purple tongue with fissures and yellow greasy fur (Fig.3.2.3.8a), short deep and faint pulse of the left hand, deep replete pulse of the right hand, and slightly weak chi-pulse. Blood routine test: WBC 4.2×10^9/L, Hb 12g/L, PLT 68×10^9/L. Gastroscopy: chronic superficial gastritis.

西医诊断：慢性浅表性胃炎。

Western medicine diagnosis: chronic superficial gastritis.

中医诊断：嘈杂。

TCM diagnosis: epigastric upset.

辨证：脾胃虚弱，中焦不运证。

Syndrome differentiation: deficiency of spleen and stomach, dysfunction of the middle energizer in transportation.

治疗：益气健脾和胃。

Treatment: replenishing qi, invigorating spleen and harmonizing stomach.

处方：香砂六君子汤加减：黄芪 15g，党参 15g，炒白术 15g，茯苓 15g，怀山药 20g，白扁豆 10g，当归 10g，丹参 15g，砂仁 6g，木香 6g。7 剂，日 1 剂，水煎服。

Prescription: modified *Xiangsha Liujunzi* Decoction.

Huangqi 15g, dangshen 15g, chaobaizhu 15g, fuling 15g, huaishanyao 20g, baibiandou 10g, danggui 10g, danshen 15g, sharen 6g, muxiang 6g.

Seven doses and one dose a day, decoction.

证候分析：脾胃虚弱，中气不足，升降失司，胃气不和而致脘闷嘈杂；食后脾气得助，则嘈杂减轻；脾胃虚弱，气血生成不足，脏腑形体失养，则神疲乏力，形体消瘦；脉道不充，则左脉短沉微，右脉沉实，尺部微弱；心神失养，则失眠；舌淡紫伴裂纹、苔黄腻，兼脉沉弱，为脾胃不足之象。

Syndrome analysis: deficiency of spleen and stomach and insufficiency of middle qi causes dysfunction of ascending and descending and disharmony of stomach qi, which leads to epigastric upset and stuffiness. Spleen qi is supported after eating, so the upset is relieved. Deficiency of spleen and stomach induces insufficient generation and transformation of qi and blood and insufficient nourishment of *zang-fu* organs, which leads to fatigue and emaciation. Unfilled vessels explain short deep and faint pulse of the left hand, deep replete pulse of the right hand, and slightly weak chi-pulse. Insufficient nourishment of the heart spirit causes insomnia. Pale purple tongue with fissures and yellow greasy fur and deep weak pulse indicate deficiency of spleen and stomach.

2017 年 5 月 17 日二诊：胃脘嘈杂不适减轻，偶有嗳气，无反酸，寐差，二便平，舌淡紫，苔薄白（图 3.2.3.8b），脉沉。原方加黄连 6g、吴茱萸 1g、珍珠母 30g，7 剂，巩固治疗。

Second visit on May 17, 2017: epigastric upset was relieved, and the patient had occasional belching without acid regurgitation, poor sleep, normal urine and stool, pale purple tongue with thin white fur (Fig.3.2.3.8b), and deep pulse. Seven doses of the previous prescription were administered to consolidate the curative effect, with the addition of huanglian 6g, wuzhuyu 1g, and zhenzhumu 30g.

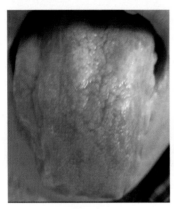 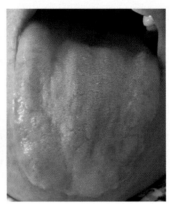

图 3.2.3.8a   图 3.2.3.8b
Fig.3.2.3.8a   Fig.3.2.3.8b

（九）腹泻 – 气虚外感证

3.9　Diarrhea: syndrome of qi deficiency and external contraction

患者杨某，女，22 岁，腹泻 3 天，于 2016 年 3 月 4 日就诊。

Patient Yang, female, 22 years old, had been suffering from diarrhea for 3 days and came to visit the doctor on March 4, 2016.

患者于 3 天前感寒湿而腹泻，日 10 余次，便溏但排出不畅，色黄，无黏液及脓血便，腹胀腹痛，肠鸣不甚，口淡不渴，纳食减少，寐可，舌质淡，苔白（图 3.2.3.9a），脉沉涩。

The patient had diarrhea more than ten times a day due to external contraction of cold-dampness three days ago. She had loose stool with unsmooth defecation and the stool was yellow without mucus, pus and blood. Moreover, she felt distending pain in the abdomen, moderate borborygmus, bland taste in the mouth without thirst, reduced appetite, normal sleep, pale tongue with white fur (Fig.3.2.3.9a), and deep unsmooth pulse.

西医诊断：腹泻。

Western medicine diagnosis: diarrhea.

中医诊断：泄泻。

TCM diagnosis: diarrhea.

辨证：寒湿困脾证。

Syndrome differentiation: cold-dampness encumbering spleen.

治疗：温中燥湿，健脾止泄。

Treatment: warming the middle and drying dampness, invigorating spleen and checking diarrhea.

处方：胃苓汤加减：炒苍术 15g，厚朴 10g，炒白术 15g，茯苓 15g，猪苓 15g，泽泻 10g，麦芽 20g，白豆蔻 15g，五味子 15g，肉桂 3g，生姜 3 片，大枣 5 枚。5 剂，日 1 剂，水煎服。

Prescription: modified *Weiling* Decoction.

Chaocangzhu 15g, houpo 10g, chaobaizhu 15g, fuling 15g, zhuling 15g, zexie 10g, maiya 20g, baidoukou 15g, wuweizi 15g, rougui 3g, shengjiang 3 pieces, dazao 5 pieces.

Five doses and one dose a day, decoction.

证候分析：外感寒湿之邪，内聚肠胃，损伤脾胃，使胃肠升降失职，清浊不分，而发生泄泻；脾胃升降失职，运化不及，则纳食减少；寒湿内侵，津液不伤，则口淡不渴；舌质淡，苔白，脉沉涩，为寒湿内阻，气血运行不及之征象。

Syndrome analysis: external contraction of cold-dampness, which accumulates in the stomach and intestine and damages the spleen and stomach, causes the stomach and intestine failing to ascend and descend and to separate lucid from turbidity, so there is diarrhea. Disorder of the ascending and descending function as well as dysfunction in transportation and transformation of spleen and stomach causes reduced appetite. Internal invasion of cold-dampness doesn't damage the body fluid, so bland taste in the mouth without thirst occurs. Pale tongue with white fur and deep unsmooth pulse are typical manifestations of internal invasion of cold-dampness and inhibited circulation of qi and blood.

2016 年 3 月 8 日二诊：大便次数明显减少，每日 3 ～ 4 次，腹胀好转，舌淡红，苔薄白（图 3.2.3.9b），脉细。继守前方 3 剂，后用归脾汤善后。

Second visit on March 8, 2016: diarrhea frequency was decreased significantly to 3-4 times a day, and abdominal distention was relieved. The patient had pale red tongue with thin white fur (Fig.3.2.3.9b), and thready pulse. Three doses of the previous prescription were administered for treatment, and after that *Guipi* Decoction was used for rehabilitation.

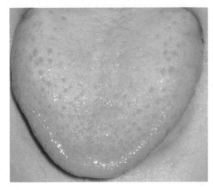 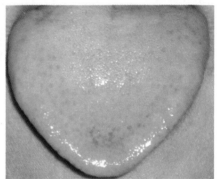

图 3.2.3.9a   图 3.2.3.9b

Fig.3.2.3.9a   Fig.3.2.3.9b

（十）便秘 – 阳虚证

3.10　Constipation: syndrome of yang deficiency

患者张某，男，68 岁，腹胀便秘 5 日，于 2011 年 9 月 20 日就诊。

Patient Zhang, male, 68 years old, had been suffering from abdominal distension and constipation for 5 days and came to visit the doctor on September 20, 2011.

患者便秘 3 年余，间断用开塞露、麻子仁丸解便，但停药后，便秘又如前。此次患者已 5 日未解大便，遂来就诊。刻诊：焦虑貌，面色㿠白，小便清长，伴腹胀纳呆，呕呃，头晕乏力，脘腹冷痛，得温痛减，喜食热饮，舌质暗淡、苔薄白（图 3.2.3.10a），脉沉迟。

The patient had been suffering from constipation for more than 3 years, with intermittent use of enema glycerin and *Maziren* Pill for smooth defecation. After stopping the drugs, the symptom was as before. He came to see the doctor due to constipation for 5 days. Present symptoms: anxious appearance, bright white complexion, profuse clear urine, abdominal distention and anorexia, vomiting and hiccup, dizziness and lassitude, epigastric and abdominal cold pain that relieves with warmth, preference for hot drinks, dark tongue with thin white fur (Fig.3.2.3.10a), and deep slow pulse.

西医诊断：习惯性便秘。

Western medicine diagnosis: habitual constipation.

中医诊断：便秘。

TCM diagnosis: constipation.

辨证：脾阳亏虚证。

Syndrome differentiation: spleen yang deficiency.

治疗：温阳健脾，润肠通便。

Treatment: warming yang and invigorating spleen, moistening intestines to relieve constipation.

处方：温脾汤加减：党参 15g，生白术 25g，熟地黄 10g，当归 10g，附子 8g（先煎），肉苁蓉 12g，干姜 6g，肉桂 3g，甘草 3g。7 剂，日 1 剂，水煎服。

Prescription: modified *Wenpi* Decoction.

Dangshen 15g, shengbaizhu 25g, shudihuang 10g, danggui 10g, fuzi 8g (decocted first), roucongrong 12g, ganjiang 6g, rougui 3g, gancao 3g.

Seven doses and one dose a day, decoction.

证候分析：脾肾阳虚，运化、排泄二便功能失职，则大便秘结，小便清长；脾肾阳虚，阴寒内盛，不能温煦全身，气机凝滞，故腹中冷痛；阳虚水泛，则面色㿠白；清阳不升，则头晕乏力；舌质淡紫、苔薄白，为脾肾阳虚，津液输布障碍，大肠传导失司之征；脉沉迟，为阳虚水寒内停之象。

Syndrome analysis: yang deficiency of spleen and kidney causes dysfunction of transportation and transformation as well as excretion, which leads to constipation and profuse clear urine. Yang deficiency of spleen and kidney with internal exuberance of yin cold fails to warm the whole body and causes stagnation of qi movement, so abdominal cold pain occurs. Yang deficiency with overflowing of water explains bright white complexion. Lucid yang failing to ascend causes dizziness and lassitude. Pale purple tongue with thin white fur is typical manifestation of yang deficiency of spleen and kidney, transmission and spreading disorder of body fluid, and conveyance disorder of large intestine. Deep slow pulse reflects yang deficiency and internal retention of water-cold.

2011 年 9 月 27 日二诊：服药后患者大便通畅，1～2 日一行，便软成形，腹中觉暖，腹胀减轻，头晕乏力症状缓解，舌质淡，苔薄黄白相间（图 3.2.3.10b），脉缓有力。以归脾汤善后。

Second visit on September 27, 2011: after taking medicine, the patient had smooth formed stool with defecation once or twice a day, and warm sensation in the abdomen. Abdominal distention, dizziness and lassitude were relieved. The tongue was pale with thin yellow and white fur (Fig.3.2.3.10b), and the pulse was moderate and forceful. *Guipi* Decoction was prescribed for rehabilitation.

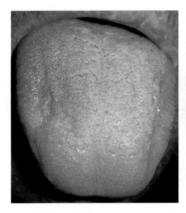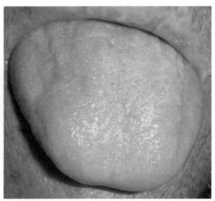

图 3.2.3.10a
Fig.3.2.3.10a

图 3.2.3.10b
Fig.3.2.3.10b

（十一）呃逆 – 气虚证

3.11 Hiccup: qi deficiency symptom

患者吴某，女，49 岁，反复呃逆 2 月余，于 2015 年 6 月 12 日就诊。

Patient Wu, female, 49 years old, had been suffering from repeated hiccup for more than 2 months and came to visit the doctor on June 12, 2015.

患者呃逆 2 月余，曾中西药物治疗，效果欠佳，为求进一步治疗而就诊。刻诊：腹满胀闷，无腹痛，纳差，食入难消，时时噫气，倦怠乏力，口淡不渴，寐可，二便可，舌质暗淡，苔白厚腻（图 3.2.3.11a），脉濡缓。

The patient had been suffering from hiccup for more than 2 months and was treated by Chinese and Western medicine without obvious efficacy, therefore she visited the doctor. Present symptoms: abdominal fullness, distention and stuffiness, no abdominal pain, poor appetite with indigestion and frequent belching, lassitude, bland taste in the mouth without thirst, normal sleep, normal urine and stool, dark pale tongue with white thick and greasy fur (Fig.3.2.3.11a), and soggy moderate pulse.

中医诊断：呃逆。

TCM diagnosis: hiccup.

辨证：胃失和降证。

Syndrome differentiation: stomach qi disharmony.

治疗：和胃降逆，调理气机。

Treatment: harmonizing stomach and descending adverse qi, regulating qi movement.

处方：旋覆代赭汤加减：旋覆花 10g（包煎），代赭石 30g（先煎），党参 12g，法半夏 10g，炒白术 15g，茯苓 15g，竹茹 12g，生姜 3 片，大枣 3 枚，谷芽 15g，炙甘草 3g。5 剂，日 1 剂，水煎服。

Prescription: modified *Xuanfu Daizhe* Decoction.

Xuanfuhua 10g (wrap-boiling), daizheshi 30g (decocted first), danshen 12g, fabanxia 10g, chaobaizhu 15g, fuling 15g, zhuru 12g, shengjiang 3 pieces, dazao 3 pieces, guya 15g, zhigancao 3g.

Five doses and one dose a day, decoction.

证候分析：脾胃虚弱，中焦气机升降运化失职，则腹满胀闷、纳差；胃气不降而上逆，则噫气频作；脾胃虚弱，气血生化不足，脏腑形体失养，则倦怠乏力；脾虚不运，津液不伤，则口淡不渴；舌质暗淡，苔白厚腻，脉濡缓，为气虚运化不足的表现。

Syndrome analysis: deficiency of spleen and stomach causes dysfunction of the middle energizer and disorder of qi movement, which leads to abdominal fullness, distention and stuffiness, and poor appetite. Stomach qi failing to descend causes frequent belching. Deficiency of spleen and stomach induces insufficient generation and transformation of qi and blood and insufficient nourishment of *zang-fu* organs, thus lassitude occurs. Spleen deficiency failing to transport and non-impairment of body fluid explains bland taste in the mouth without thirst. Dark pale tongue with white thick and greasy fur and soggy moderate pulse indicate qi deficiency and insufficient transportation and transformation.

2015 年 6 月 17 日二诊：患者呃逆明显减轻、纳食可，脘腹胀减轻，胃气有下降之势，舌质淡红，苔薄白（图 3.2.3.11b），脉弦。效不更方，继服前方 5 剂而愈。

Second visit on June 17, 2015: hiccup was significantly reduced and abdominal distention was relieved with stomach qi descending. The patient had normal appetite, pale red tongue with thin white fur (Fig.3.2.3.11b), and wiry pulse. Five doses of the previous prescription were used for treatment.

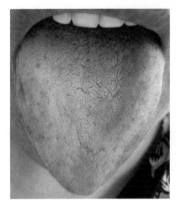
图 3.2.3.11a
Fig.3.2.3.11a

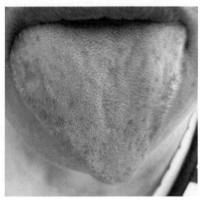
图 3.2.3.11b
Fig.3.2.3.11b

（十二）呕吐 – 肝气犯胃证

3.12 Vomiting: syndrome of liver qi invading stomach

患者章某，男，56 岁，呕吐 1 周加重 3 天，于 2013 年 4 月 13 日就诊。

Patient Zhang, male, 56 years old, had been suffering from vomiting for one week and the symptoms aggravated 3 days ago. So he came to visit the doctor on April 13, 2013.

患者 1 周前因家庭关系不睦而情志不舒，饮食减少，胸闷嗳气，后出现恶心呕吐，食后即吐，吐后觉舒，曾肌注胃复安，呕吐症状减轻，继而又吐，吐出清水或食物，胁肋胀闷，头昏脑涨，寐可，二便平，舌暗红，苔白腻（图 3.2.3.12a），脉弦。消化道造影（－）。

The patient suffered from emotional discomfort due to inharmonious family relations one week ago, with reduced appetite, chest stuffiness, belching, nausea and vomiting that features immediate vomiting of ingested food and subjective comfort after vomiting. The patient was injected with metoclopramide and vomiting was relieved. But he continued to vomit clear water or food, with hypochondriac distention and stuffiness, dizziness and heavy feeling in the brain, normal sleep, normal urine and stool, dark red tongue with white greasy fur (Fig.3.2.3.12a), and wiry pulse. Gastrointestinal imaging (-).

西医诊断：胃炎。

Western medicine diagnosis: gastritis.

中医诊断：呕吐。

TCM diagnosis: vomiting.

辨证：肝气犯胃，胃气上逆证。

Syndrome differentiation: liver qi invading stomach, stomach qi ascending counterflow.

治疗：疏肝理气，降逆止呕。

Treatment: soothing liver and regulating qi, descending counterflow of qi and arresting vomiting.

处方：旋覆代赭汤加减：柴胡 10g，香附 8g，法半夏 10g，陈皮 8g，旋覆花 15g（包煎），代赭石 20g（先煎），茯苓 15g，白术 15g，竹茹 10g，麦芽 10g，夜交藤 30g，玫瑰花 10g。5 剂，日 1 剂，水煎服。

Prescription: modified *Xuanfu Daizhe* Decoction.

Chaihu 10g, xiangfu 8g, fabanxia 10g, chenpi 8g, xuanfuhua 15g (wrap-boiling), daizheshi 20g (decocted first), fuling 15g, baizhu 15g, zhuru 10g, maiya 10g, yejiaoteng 30g, meiguihua 10g.

Five doses and one dose a day, decoction.

证候分析：肝调畅情志，主疏泄，肝气郁结，疏泄失职，则胁肋胀闷；肝气横逆犯胃，胃失和降，胃气上逆，则恶心呕吐，嗳气频作；胃气不降，脾气不升，则头昏脑涨；中焦气机受阻，则纳食不进；舌暗红，苔白腻，脉弦，为肝气犯胃之明证。

Syndrome analysis: the liver's physiological function is to regulate emotions and govern free coursing. Liver qi depression causes dysfunction of free coursing, therefore, hypochondriac distention and stuffiness occurs. Liver qi transversely invading stomach causes disharmony of stomach qi and stomach qi ascending counterflow, which leads to nausea and vomiting, frequent belching. Stomach qi failing to descend and spleen qi failing to ascend brings dizziness and heavy feeling in the brain. Qi obstruction in the middle energizer causes poor appetite. Dark red tongue with white greasy fur and wiry pulse are obvious manifestations of liver qi invading stomach.

2013 年 4 月 18 日二诊：患者诉呕吐明显减轻，胁肋胀痛好转，寐可，纳差，舌淡，苔白（图 3.2.3.12b）。原方减竹茹，加麦芽 20g、神曲 20g，继服 5 剂。

Second visit on April 18, 2013: vomiting was significantly reduced and hypochondriac distention and stuffiness was relieved. The patient had normal sleep, poor appetite, pale tongue with white fur (Fig.3.2.3.12b). Five doses of the previous prescription were used for treatment, with the reduction of zhuru and the addition of maiya 20g, shenqu 20g.

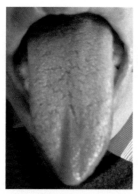 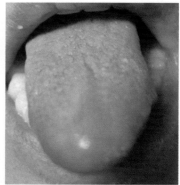

图 3.2.3.12a   图 3.2.3.12b
Fig.3.2.3.12a   Fig.3.2.3.12b

四、肺系病证

4. Respiratory disease syndrome

（一）咳嗽 – 风寒袭肺证

4.1　Cough: syndrome of wind-cold fettering lung

患者徐某，女，47 岁，咳嗽 1 月余加重 5 天，于 2016 年 4 月 2 日就诊。

Patient Xu, female, 47 years old, had been suffering from cough for more than one month and the symptom aggravated five days ago, so she visited the doctor on

April 2, 2016.

患者于 1 个月前因受寒感冒伴咳嗽，咳白色泡沫痰，经中西医治疗感冒好转而咳嗽不减，5 天前继续输液治疗，症状不减，遂来就诊。刻诊：咳嗽声哑，痰出而黏白，胸胁胀满，夜寐不能平卧，左肺底可闻及少量肺泡音，纳食可，寐差，二便平，舌质淡，苔白稍腻（图 3.2.4.1a），脉沉。

The patient had a common cold and coughed up white foam phlegm. After the treatment of Chinese and Western medicine, the common cold was improved except cough that was further treated by infusion therapy 5 days ago, but the symptoms had not improved. Therefore she came to see the doctor. Present symptoms: cough, hoarse voice, sticky white phlegm, fullness in chest and hypochondrium, inability to lie flat when sleeping at night, few alveolar sounds at the bottom of the left lung, normal appetite, poor sleep, normal urine and stool, pale tongue with white greasy fur (Fig.3.2.4.1a), and deep pulse.

中医诊断：咳嗽。

TCM diagnosis: cough.

辨证：风寒束肺证。

Syndrome differentiation: wind-cold fettering lung.

治疗：宣肺解表，降逆止咳。

Treatment: dispersing lung and relieving exterior, descending adverse qi and relieving cough.

处方：苏子降气汤加减：紫苏子 15g，杏仁 10g，桔梗 10g，木蝴蝶 15g，五味子 10g，前胡 10g，厚朴 10g，茯苓 12g，浙贝母 10g，生姜 3 片，大枣 3 枚。3 剂，日 1 剂，水煎服。

Prescription: modified *Suzi Jiangqi* Decoction.

Zisuzi 15g, xingren 10g, jiegeng 10g, muhudie 15g, wuweizi 10g, qianhu 10g, houpo 10g, fuling 12g, zhebeimu 10g, shengjiang 3 pieces, dazao 3 pieces.

Three doses and one dose a day, decoction.

证候分析：风寒束肺，宣降失职，水津不布，酿生痰浊，阻滞肺窍，出现咳白色泡沫痰、咳嗽声哑、胸胁胀满等症；舌质淡、苔白腻，提示寒湿内蕴，脉沉主里证。

Syndrome analysis: wind-cold fettering lung causes the lung's dysfunction in dispersing and descending and the abnormal transformation of water-fluid, which produces phlegm-turbidity that obstructs the lung. Therefore, the symptoms such as cough with white foam phlegm, hoarse voice, and fullness in chest and hypochondrium appear. Pale tongue and white-greasy fur suggest internal accumulation of cold-dampness while deep pulse is the sign of interior syndrome.

2016 年 4 月 5 日二诊：患者自诉服药当晚咳嗽明显减轻，能平卧，寐可，唯口干明显，舌质淡红、苔白而干（图 3.2.4.1b），脉沉。治以养阴润肺，生津止咳。方用桑杏汤善后。

Second visit on April 5, 2016: the patient told that she could lie flat with cough alleviated after medication at the very night. Present symptoms: cough and expectoration were improved markedly, normal sleep, only obvious dry mouth, pink tongue with white dry fur (Fig.3.2.4.1b), and deep pulse. Treatment: nourishing yin and moistening lung, promoting fluid production to quench thirst. *Sangxin* Decoction was used for treatment.

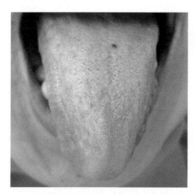 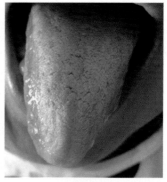

图 3.2.4.1a   图 3.2.4.1b

Fig.3.2.4.1a   Fig.3.2.4.1b

（二）咳嗽 – 痰湿壅肺证

4.2　Cough: syndrome of phlegm-dampness obstructing lung

患者马某，女，63 岁，咳嗽咯痰 10 月余伴痰中带血 10 余天，于 2017 年 4 月 29 日就诊。

Patient Ma, female, 63 years old, had been suffering from cough and expectoration for more than 10 months. In recent 10 days, there was blood in the phlegm, so she came to visit the doctor on April 29, 2017.

患者 10 个月前无明显诱因出现咳嗽，咽痒即咳，行胸部 CT 片示左肺下叶条索状影，拟慢性炎症改变，曾口服药物治疗，但症状持续不减。10 天前患者无明显诱因咳嗽咯痰加重伴痰中带血，为求进一步治疗前来医院就诊。刻诊：恶风，自汗，口干，颈项强直，咳嗽咳痰，咳嗽阵作，咳白脓痰，不易咳出，夜寐欠佳，纳食尚可，小便调，大便先干后稀，舌质暗淡，苔白而腻（图 3.2.4.2a），脉濡。肺部 CT 示：前纵隔胸腺区占位，考虑侵袭性腺瘤；肺气肿；左肺上叶与右肺下叶结节影，拟为良性稳定性病变；左肺下叶肺气囊；双侧锁骨下肿大淋巴结。肺功能示：重度阻塞性通气功能障碍；肺气肿；肺弥漫性功能正常。

The patient had cough without obvious reason 10 months ago, especially when the pharyngeal was itching. Chest CT showed chronic inflammation change with stripe-like shadow in the inferior lobe of left lung, and oral administration didn't work well. Ten days ago, cough and expectoration of blood-stained phlegm became serious without obvious cause. For further treatment, she came to see the doctor. Present symptoms: aversion to wind, spontaneous sweating, dry mouth, rigid neck, cough and expectoration, paroxysmal cough with white purulent phlegm that was difficult to expectorate, poor sleep, normal appetite, normal urine, dry stool followed by loose one, dark pale tongue with white greasy fur (Fig.3.2.4.2a), and soggy pulse. Lung CT: aggressive adenoma with the anterior mediastinal thymus occupied; emphysema; nodular shadow in the upper lobe of left lung and the inferior lobe of right lung, which was diagnosed as benign stable lesion; air sacs in the inferior lobe of left lung; bilateral subclavian lymphadenectasis. Lung function: severe obstructive ventilation dysfunction; emphysema; normal pulmonary diffuse function.

既往史：慢性胃炎病史 10 余年，胆囊切除手术史 5 年。

Past medical history: chronic gastritis for more than 10 years, cholecystecyomy for 5 years.

西医诊断：肺部感染；慢性胃炎；胆囊切除术后状态。

Western medicine diagnosis: pulmonary infection; chronic gastritis; status after cholecystectomy.

中医诊断：咳嗽。

TCM diagnosis: cough.

辨证：痰湿阻肺证。

Syndrome differentiation: phlegm-dampness obstructing lung.

治疗：健脾利湿，化痰止咳。

Treatment: invigorating spleen and draining dampness, resolving phlegm and relieving cough.

处方：四君子汤加减：党参10g，炒白术15g，苍术10g，茯苓15g，橘络8g，乌梅10g，鱼腥草20g，桔梗10g，杏仁10g，白花蛇舌草20g，石见穿15g，紫菀10g，生姜3片。7剂，日1剂，水煎服。

Prescription: modified *Sijunzi* Decoction.

Dangshen 10g, chaobaizhu 15g, cangzhu 10g, fuling 15g, juluo 8g, wumei 10g, yuxingcao 20g, jiegeng 10g, xingren 10g, baihuasheshecao 20g, shijianchuan 15g, ziwan 10g, shengjiang 3 pieces.

Seven doses and one dose a day, decoction.

证候分析：久病咳嗽，耗伤气阴，肺气不足，子盗母气，致脾气亏虚，运化失职，酿生痰浊，上贮于肺，而见咳嗽咳痰，咳嗽阵作，咳白脓痰；久咳伤肺，肺络损伤，而见痰中带血；舌暗淡、苔白而腻；咳脓白痰，不易咳出，提示痰湿阻于肺系。

Syndrome analysis: chronic cough results in the damage of qi and yin. Deficiency of lung qi causes insufficiency of spleen qi because disorder of child-organ affects mother-organ. Insufficiency of spleen qi with dysfunction in transportation and transformation produces phlegm and turbidity that are stored upward in the lung. Therefore, such symptoms as expectoration and paroxysmal cough with white purulent phlegm appear. Prolonged cough damaging lung collaterals brings about bloody phlegm. Dark pale tongue with white greasy fur and white purulent phlegm that was difficult to expectorate suggest phlegm-dampness obstructing lung.

2017年5月6日二诊：患者精神可，咳嗽症状减轻，偶有痰中带血，痰量少，夜寐不佳，大小便正常，舌淡红、苔薄白（图3.2.4.2b），脉缓。原方加夜交藤30g、合欢皮20g，7剂。嘱患者定期检查，以排除占位性病变。

Second visit on May 6, 2017: the patient had normal spirit, relieved cough, small amount of occasional bloody phlegm, poor sleep, normal urine and stool, pale red tongue with thin white fur (Fig.3.2.4.2b), and moderate pulse. Seven doses of the previous prescription were used for treatment, with the addition of yejiaoteng 30g and hehuanpi 20g. The patient was advised to examine the body regularly to exclude space occupying lesions.

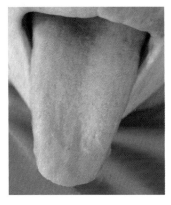

图 3.2.4.2a
Fig.3.2.4.2a

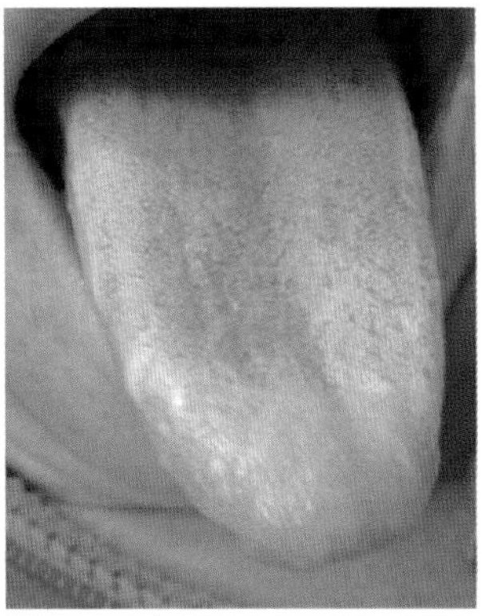

图 3.2.4.2b
Fig.3.2.4.2b

（三）咳嗽 – 痰热壅肺证

4.3 Cough: syndrome of phlegm-heat obstructing lung

患者秦某，男，69 岁，咳嗽 10 余天，发热 2 天，于 2017 年 4 月 22 日就诊。

Patient Qin, male, 69 years old, had been suffering from cough for more than 10 days and fever for 2 days. So he came to visit the doctor on April 22, 2017.

患者 10 天前受凉后出现咳嗽，鼻塞流涕，未系统治疗，昨日出现恶寒、体温升高，经当地医院治疗体温有所下降，仍咳嗽，咳少量白黏痰，为求进一步求治而来就诊。刻诊：咳嗽，咳少量白黏痰，晨起流清涕且咳少量黄痰，难以咳出，口干夜甚，发热，盗汗，口唇稍发绀，左侧偏瘫，行动不利，夜寐差，纳食减，二便调，舌质暗红，苔黄腻（图 3.2.4.3a），脉弦滑偏数。血常规检查示：考虑感染。肺部 CT 示：双肺散在条索影、斑片影，拟感染改变。

Ten days ago, the patient had cough, nasal congestion and runny nose after cold attack, without systematic treatment. He felt aversion to cold and rising temperature yesterday. After the treatment in the local hospital, body temperature was dropped but the patient still had cough with scanty white sticky phlegm. For further treatment, he came to see the doctor. Present symptoms: cough and expectoration of scanty white sticky phlegm, clear snivel in the morning get-up time with difficult expectoration of scanty yellow phlegm, dry mouth that got worse at night, fever, night sweat, slightly cyanotic lips, hemiplegia in left side with difficult movement, poor sleep, reduced appetite, normal urine and stool, dark red tongue with yellow greasy fur (Fig.3.2.4.3a), and wiry slippery and slightly rapid pulse. Blood routine test: infection. Pulmonary CT: infected change with interspersed linear opacities and patchy shadows.

既往史：高血压病史 10 余年，中风病史 10 余年，有结核病史。

Past Medical History: tuberculosis; more than 10 years of hypertension and wind stroke.

西医诊断：肺部感染；高血压Ⅲ期；脑梗死后遗症；全身性骨关节炎。

Western medicine diagnosis: pulmonary infection; hypertension (phase Ⅲ); sequelae of cerebral infarction; systemic osteoarthritis.

中医诊断：咳嗽。

TCM diagnosis: cough.

辨证：痰热壅肺证。

Syndrome differentiation: phlegm-heat obstructing lung.

治疗：清热化痰，肃肺止咳。

Treatment: clearing heat and resolving phlegm, astringing lung and relieving cough.

处方：麻杏石甘汤加减：生石膏 30g，北沙参 30g，黄芩 10g，麻黄 6g，杏仁 10g，百部 10g，紫菀 10g，射干 10g，浙贝母 10g，紫苏子 10g，地龙 10g，枇杷叶 10g，生甘草 3g。7 剂，日 1 剂，水煎服。

Prescription: modified *Maxing Shigan* Decoction.

Shengshigao 30g, beishashen 30g, huangqin 10g, mahuang 6g, xingren 10g, baibu 10g, ziyuan 10g, zhebeimu 10g, zisuzi 10g, dilong 10g, pipaye 10g, shenggancao 3g.

Seven doses and one dose a day, decoction.

证候分析：外感风寒束肺，肺失宣降而出现咳嗽、咳痰清稀；治疗不及时，寒邪有郁而化热之象，故出现晨起咳少量黄痰；苔黄腻，提示有湿热之征；脉弦滑偏数，佐证湿热内阻的存在。

Syndrome analysis: wind-cold fettering lung and lung qi failing in dispersing and descending result in cough with clear phlegm. Delayed treatment causes depressed cold pathogen transforming into heat, which causes expectoration of scanty yellow phlegm in the morning get-up time. Yellow greasy fur suggests dampness-heat, and wiry slippery and slightly rapid pulse is the manifestation of internal obstruction of dampness-heat.

2017 年 4 月 29 日二诊：咳嗽症状明显好转，无口干、发热，舌暗红，苔白（图 3.2.4.3b），脉弦。维持原方 7 剂，巩固治疗。

Second visit on April 29, 2017: cough was improved significantly, and the patient had no dry mouth and fever, dark red tongue with white fur (Fig.3.2.4.3b), and wiry pulse. Seven doses of the previous prescription were used to consolidate the effect.

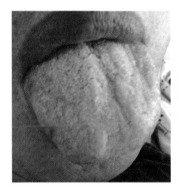 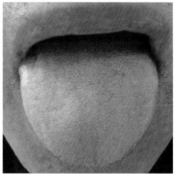

图 3.2.4.3a   图 3.2.4.3b
Fig.3.2.4.3a   Fig.3.2.4.3b

（四）喘证 – 肺气虚证

4.4　Dyspnea: syndrome of qi deficiency of lung

患者文某，女，67 岁，反复胸闷气喘、咳嗽咳痰 2 余年，再发 2 月余，于 2017 年 4 月 15 日就诊。

Patient Wen, female, 67 years old, had been suffering from recurrent chest oppression, dyspnea, cough and expectoration for more than 2 years. She came to visit the doctor on April 15, 2017 because of its recurrence for more than 2 months.

患者 2 年前因劳累后出现胸闷气喘、咳嗽咳痰，未系统治疗，之后症状每于冬春季受凉而诱发，行间断治疗。近 2 月来，患者受凉后胸闷气喘、咳嗽咳痰症状加重，遂来就诊。刻诊：胸闷气喘，上二楼即喘，气短不足以息，咳嗽咳痰，痰色白，每天十余口，胸背部游走性疼痛，乏力易累，平素怕冷易感，口干喜热饮，夜间甚，嗝声连连，饮水、进食易呛，无咽喉不适，无鼻塞流涕，无头晕头痛，无腹胀腹痛，纳食可，夜寐差，二便调。舌质暗红，苔黄腻（图 3.2.4.4a），脉沉。血气分析示：酸碱度7.41，二氧化碳分压 38mmHg，氧分压 271mmHg，碳酸氢根 24.1mmol/L，氧饱和度 100%。血常规检查示：白细胞 3.71×10^9/L，血红蛋白 106g/L。

The patient suffered from chest oppression, dyspnea, cough and expectoration due to fatigue 2 years ago, without systematic treatment. From then on, the symptoms were triggered by cold attack in winter and spring, with intermittent treatment. In recent 2 months, the syndromes of chest oppression, dyspnea, cough and expectoration got worse after cold attack, so she came to see the doctor. Present symptoms: chest oppression, dyspnea (even climbing the second floor), shortness of breath, cough with expectoration of more than 10 mouthful white phlegm a day, migratory pain in chest and back, fatigue, easy tiredness, fear of cold, susceptible to cold, dry mouth with preference to hot drink that got worse at night, frequent hiccup, easily to be chocked while drinking and eating, no throat discomfort, no nasal congestion and runny nose, no dizziness and headache, no abdominal distension and pain, normal appetite, poor sleep, normal urine and stool, dark red tongue with yellow greasy fur (Fig.3.2.4.4a), and deep pulse. Arterial blood gas analysis: pH 7.41, partial pressure of carbon dioxide 38 mmHg, partial pressure of oxygen271mmHg, T bicarbonate radical 24.1mmol/L, oxygen saturation 100%. Blood routine test: WBC 3.71×10^9/L, Hb 106g/L.

既往史：既往有慢性萎缩性胃炎病史，否认高血压、糖尿病、心脏病史，否认肝炎、结核病史，有剖宫产史，无重大外伤史，有输血史，预防接种史不详。

Past medical history: chronic atrophic gastritis; denied diseases of hypertension, diabetes, heart disease, hepatitis, tuberculosis, and severe trauma; cesarean section, blood transfusion; unknown vaccination history.

西医诊断：慢性支气管炎；慢性胃炎。

Western medicine diagnosis: chronic bronchitis; chronic gastritis.

中医诊断：喘证。

TCM diagnosis: dyspnea syndrome.

辨证：肺脾气虚证。

Syndrome differentiation: qi deficiency of lung and spleen.

治疗：健脾益气，化痰止咳。

Treatment: invigorating spleen and replenishing qi, resolving phlegm and relieving cough.

处方：健脾汤加减：党参 15g，黄芪 15g，炒白术 15g，茯苓 15g，杏仁 10g，桔梗 10g，陈皮 10g，百果 10g，款冬花 10g，紫苏子 10g，代赭石 20g，紫苏叶 10g，生姜 3 片，大枣 5 枚。7 剂，日 1 剂，水煎服。

Prescription: modified *Jianpi* Decoction.

Dangshen 15g, huangqi 15g, chaobaizhu 15g, fuling 15g, xingren 10g, jiegeng 10g, chenpi 10g, baiguo 10g, kuandonghua 15g, zisuzi 10g, daizheshi 20g, zisuye 10g, shengjiang 3 pieces, dazao 5 pieces.

Seven doses and one dose a day, decoction.

证候分析：久病体弱，脾气亏虚，母病及子，出现咳嗽咳痰，气短乏力；舌质暗为脾虚气机运行无力，致血行受阻而成瘀；舌苔黄腻，脉沉，为脾虚湿蕴之证。

Syndrome analysis: chronic disease results in weak constitution and spleen qi deficiency. So, symptoms of cough, expectoration, shortness of breath and fatigue happen because the disorder of mother-organ affects child-organ. Dark red tongue is caused by spleen deficiency and forceless propelling of qi movement that obstructs the blood movement and causes blood stasis. Yellow greasy fur and deep pulse are the manifestations of spleen deficiency with dampness retention.

2017 年 4 月 22 日二诊：咳嗽咳痰、胸闷气喘减轻，偶有呃声，寐差，余无不适，舌淡红，苔薄黄（图 3.2.4.4b），脉缓无力。原方加茯神 20g，7 剂，继续治疗。

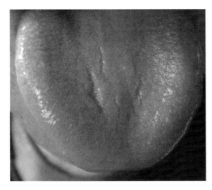 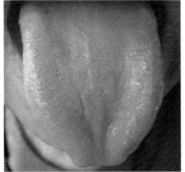

图 3.2.4.4a　　　　　　　　图 3.2.4.4b
Fig.3.2.4.4a　　　　　　　　Fig.3.2.4.4b

Second visit on April 22, 2017: the symptoms of cough, expectoration, chest oppression and dyspnea were relieved, and the patient had occasional hiccup, poor sleep, no other discomfort, pale red tongue with thin yellow fur (Fig.3.2.4.4b), and moderate weak pulse. Seven doses of the previous prescription were used for further treatment, with the addition of fushen 20g.

（五）喘证 – 痰热蕴肺证

4.5　Dyspnea: syndrome of phlegm-heat accumulating lung

患者索某，男，63 岁，间断性咳嗽、喘憋 10 年加重伴气急不能平卧 5 天，于 2013 年 12 月 13 日就诊。

Patient Suo, male, 63 years old, had been suffering from intermittent cough and asthma for 10 years, and the symptoms got worse with dyspnea and inability to lie flat for 5 days. So he came to visit the doctor on December 13, 2013.

刻诊：咳嗽胸闷，咳痰黄稠难出，呈端坐位，口唇青紫，颈静脉怒张，双下肢轻度浮肿，口渴而不欲饮，口中黏腻，纳差，寐差，二便平，舌质暗红，苔黄厚腻（图 3.2.4.5a），脉滑数。听诊：两肺可闻及痰鸣音，双下肺可闻及湿啰音。心率 98 次 / 分，律齐。

Present symptoms: chest oppression, cough with difficult expectoration of thick yellow phlegm, keeping sitting position, cyanotic lips, cervical venous engorgement, slight edema of lower limbs, thirst without desire to drink, sticky and greasy sensation in the mouth, poor appetite and sleep, normal urine and stool, dark red tongue with yellow thick and greasy fur (Fig.3.2.4.5a), and slippery rapid pulse. Auscultation: phlegm-gurgling sounds in both lungs, and wet rales in both lower lungs. Heart rate: 98 times per minute, normal cardiac rhythm.

西医诊断：慢性支气管炎继发肺部感染。

Western medicine diagnosis: chronic bronchitis and secondary pulmonary infection.

中医诊断：喘证。

TCM diagnosis: dyspnea syndrome.

辨证：湿热内阻，肺窍失宣证。

Syndrome differentiation: internal obstruction of dampness-heat, failure of lung to disperse.

处方：小陷胸汤加减：瓜蒌 30g，法半夏 10g，黄连 6g，厚朴 10g，杏仁 10g，桔梗 10g，紫苏子 10g，款冬花 10g，茯苓 15g，川贝母 10g，大腹皮 10g。7 剂，日 1 剂，水煎服。

Prescription: modified *Xiaoxianxiong* Decoction.

Gualou 30g, fabanxia 10g, huanglian 6g, houpo 10g, xingren 10g, jiegeng 10g, zisuzi 10g, kuandonghua 10g, fuling 15g, chuanbeimu 10g, dafupi 10g.

Seven doses and one dose a day, decoction.

证候分析：湿热内蕴于肺，肺气不利，肺失宣降，则咳嗽胸闷，咳痰；湿性黏滞，则咳痰难出；湿热阻滞，则口渴而不欲饮，口中黏腻；湿热阻滞，气血运行不畅，则舌质暗红；苔黄厚腻，脉滑数，为湿热内蕴之征。

Syndrome analysis: internal accumulation of dampness-heat in lung causes failure of lung to disperse and descend, which causes cough, chest oppression and expectoration. The sticky nature of dampness explains difficult expectoration. Dampness-heat obstruction leads to thirst without desire to drink, and sticky greasy sensation in the mouth. Dampness-heat obstruction generates inhibited movement of qi and blood, so dark red tongue manifests. And yellow thick and greasy fur and slippery rapid pulse indicate internal accumulation of dampness-heat.

2013 年 12 月 20 日二诊：胸闷减轻，夜寐可以平卧，两下肢水肿减轻，仍有轻微咳嗽，痰难出，舌质淡红，苔薄黄腻（图 3.2.4.5b）。原方加鲜竹沥 15g，继服 10 剂。咳嗽咳痰、胸闷等症状明显好转，两肺偶可闻及痰鸣音，无湿啰音，两下肢浮肿消失。

Second visit on December 20, 2013: chest oppression and edema of lower limbs had been alleviated. The patient could lie flat to sleep at night, and had mild cough, difficult expectoration, pale red tongue with yellow thin and greasy fur (Fig.3.2.4.5b). Ten doses of the previous prescription were still used for treatment, with the addition of xianzhuli 15g. After medication, the symptoms of cough, expectoration and chest oppression were improved significantly. Occasional phlegm-gurgling sounds could be heard in both lungs, and wet rales and edema of lower limbs were disappeared.

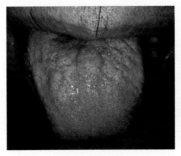 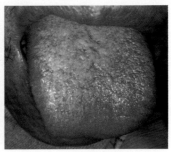

图 3.2.4.5a
Fig.3.2.4.5a

图 3.2.4.5b
Fig.3.2.4.5b

（六）哮喘 – 肺脾气虚证

4.6　Asthma: syndrome of qi deficiency of lung and spleen

患者熊某，男，52 岁，反复咳喘 30 年加重 1 月，伴双下肢浮肿 1 周，于 2017 年 4 月 23 日就诊。

Patient Xiong, male, 52 years old, had been suffering from repeated cough and asthma for 30 years. The symptoms aggravated one month ago with edema of lower limbs for one week, so he visited the doctor on April 23, 2017.

患者 30 年前无明显诱因出现咳嗽、喘息、胸闷，喉中痰鸣，休息时好转，未系统治疗。上述症状反复发作，每于冬春季节或受凉后诱发，且呈逐年加重趋势。1 月前受凉后咳嗽、喘息加重，7 天前发现双下肢轻度水肿，无力，步行困难，遂来就诊。刻诊：胸闷，气逼、气喘，喉中哮鸣音，尚可平卧，无咳嗽咳痰，咽干，口苦，恶寒，无发热，胃脘部胀闷不适，无嗳腐吞酸，无恶心呕吐，双下肢乏力，步行困难，食纳尚可，夜寐安，二便平。舌质淡红、苔白腻而水滑（图 3.2.4.6a），脉滑。

Thirty years ago, the patient suffered from cough, asthma, chest distress, and phlegm-gurgling sounds in the throat without obvious inducement. These symptoms were alleviated at rest, and he didn't receive systematic treatment. The above-mentioned symptoms recurred in winter or spring season or after cold attack, with increasing aggravation year by year. The patient had aggravated cough and asthma since cold attack one month ago, and found mild edema, weakness in the lower limbs with difficult walking 7 days ago, therefore he came to see the doctor. Present symptoms: chest distress, depression of qi, asthma, phlegm-gurgling sounds in the throat, ability to lie flat, no cough and expectoration, dry throat, bitter taste in the mouth, aversion to cold, no fever, epigastric distension and tightness, no belching and acid regurgitation, no nausea and vomiting, weakness in the lower limbs with difficult walking, normal appetite and sleep, normal urine and stool, pale red tongue with white greasy and slippery fur (Fig.3.2.4.6a), and slippery pulse.

既往史：高血压病史；慢性肺源性心脏病史。

Past medical history: hypertension; chronic pulmonary heart disease.

西医诊断：支气管哮喘；慢性阻塞性肺病伴急性加重；慢性肺源性心脏病；高血压Ⅰ期；慢性胃炎。

Western medicine diagnosis: bronchial asthma; acute aggravation of chronic obstructive pulmonary disease; chronic pulmonary heart disease; hypertension (phase Ⅰ); chronic gastritis.

中医诊断：哮喘病。

TCM diagnosis: Asthma.

辨证：肺脾气虚证。

Syndrome differentiation: qi deficiency of lung and spleen.

治疗：健脾益气，止咳平喘。

Treatment: invigorating spleen and replenishing qi, relieving cough and asthma.

处方：定喘汤加减：党参 20g，炙黄芪 15g，炒白术 15g，茯苓 15g，紫苏子 10g，炙麻黄 10g，杏仁 10g，桑白皮 15g，冬瓜子 30g ，款冬花 15g。7 剂，日 1 剂，水煎服。

Prescription: modified *Dingchuan* Decoction.

Dangshen 20g, zhihuangqi 15g, chaobaizhu 15g, fuling 15g, zisuzi 10g, zhimahuang 10g, xingren 10g, sangbaipi 15g, dongguazi 30g, kuandonghua 15g.

Seven doses and one dose a day, decoction.

证候分析：肺脾气虚，运化无力，水湿内停，生痰成饮，上贮于肺，见咳嗽，喘息，胸闷，喉中痰鸣，休息时好转；肺气不利，痰浊阻滞，而见胸闷，气逼，气喘；舌质淡，苔白腻而水滑，脉滑，为痰湿内盛的表现。

Syndrome analysis: qi deficiency of lung and spleen causes the spleen's dysfunction in transformation and transportation and internal retention of water-dampness, which produces phlegm and fluid that flow upward and are stored in the lung. Therefore, there appear cough, asthma, chest distress, and phlegm-gurgling sounds in the throat that is alleviated at rest. Inhibition of lung qi and obstruction of phlegm-turbidity causes chest distress, depression of qi, and asthma. Pale tongue with white greasy and slippery fur and slippery pulse indicate internal exuberance of phlegm-dampness.

2017 年 4 月 30 二诊：胸闷、喘息稍减，喉中偶有哮鸣音，双下肢浮肿有所减轻，舌淡，苔白腻（图 3.2.4.6b），脉滑。原方加猪苓 15g、泽泻 10g、大腹皮 15g，7 剂，维持治疗。

Second visit on April 30, 2017: chest distress and asthma were alleviated slightly, with occasional phlegm-gurgling sounds in the throat. Edema in the lower limbs was relieved, and the patient had pale tongue with white greasy fur (Fig.3.2.4.6b), and slippery pulse. Seven doses of the previous prescription were administered for treatment, with the addition of zhuling 15g, zexie 10g, and dafupi 15g.

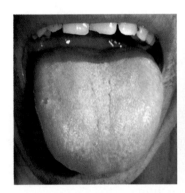 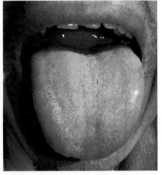

图 3.2.4.6a
Fig.3.2.4.6a

图 3.2.4.6b
Fig.3.2.4.6b

（七）哮证 – 冷哮证

4.7 Wheezing: cold wheezing syndrome

患者常某，男，51 岁，哮证发作 5 日，于 2014 年 11 月 20 日就诊。

Patient Chang, male, 51 years old, had been suffering from wheezing for 5 days, so he visited the doctor on November 20, 2014.

患者哮喘病史多年，每于秋冬天气变化时发作，每次发作均需住院输液治疗。5

日前患者因天气变化而引发哮喘，自服氨茶碱、螺旋霉素等药物，症状不减，遂来就诊。刻诊：精神不振，面色苍白，口唇发绀，胸闷气憋，喘如拉锯，夜间不能平卧，咳出少量白痰，畏寒无汗，流清涕，寐差，纳可，二便平，舌紫暗，苔白滑（图3.2.4.7a），脉弦滑。

The patient had asthma for many years, which occurred with weather change in autumn and spring, and every time he needed hospital infusion treatment. Asthma was re-induced by the change of weather 5 days ago, and he took aminophylline and spiramycin by himself without obvious efficacy. Therefore, he came to see the doctor. Present symptoms: dispiritedness, pale complexion, cyanotic lips, chest distress, depression of qi, wheezing sound, inability to lie flat at night, expectoration of scanty white phlegm, aversion to cold, adiaphoresis, clear snivel, poor sleep, normal appetite, normal urine and stool, dark purple tongue with white slippery fur (Fig.3.2.4.7a), and wiry slippery pulse.

西医诊断：哮喘。

Western medicine diagnosis: asthma.

中医诊断：哮证。

TCM diagnosis: wheezing.

辨证：风寒外束，痰饮伏肺证。

Syndrome differentiation: wind-cold fettering the exterior, latent phlegm and fluid-retention in the lung.

治疗：祛风散寒，化痰降逆。

Treatment: dispelling wind and dissipating cold, resolving phlegm and descending adverse qi.

处方：小青龙汤加减：麻黄 10g，杏仁 10g，干姜 10g，厚朴 15g，大腹皮 10g，紫苏子 10g，法半夏 10g，陈皮 6g，白果 15g，地龙 10g。7 剂，日 1 剂，水煎服。

Prescription: modified *Xiaoqinglong* Decoction.

Mahuang 10g, xingren 10g, ganjiang 10g, houpo 15g, dafupi 10g, zisuzi 10g, fabanxia 10g, chenpi 6g, baiguo 15g, dilong 10g.

Seven doses and one dose a day, decoction.

证候分析：素有哮喘，近因受寒而引动伏饮宿痰，痰随气升，壅塞气道而致胸闷气憋，喘如拉锯，咳出少量白痰；寒邪外束而见畏寒无汗，流清涕；舌紫暗，苔白腻，脉弦滑，为内有伏饮之征。

Syndrome analysis: long-term asthma and recent cold attack triggered the latent phlegm and fluid-retention to ascend with qi, which obstructs the air-way and causes chest distress, wheezing sound, and expectoration of scanty white phlegm. Wind-cold fettering the exterior causes aversion to cold, adiaphoresis and clear snivel. Dark purple tongue with white slippery fur and wiry slippery pulse suggest the latent fluid-retention.

2014 年 11 月 27 日二诊：服药后患者哮喘症状明显减轻，胸不闷，夜寐平卧，舌淡紫，苔薄白（图 3.2.4.7b），脉缓。予六君子汤善后。

Second visit on November 27, 2014: the symptoms of asthma were alleviated after taking the medicine. The patient had no chest distress, ability to lie flat at night, pale purple tongue with thin white fur (Fig.3.2.4.7b), and moderate pulse. *Liujunzi* Decoction was used for rehabilitation.

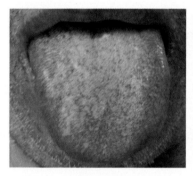 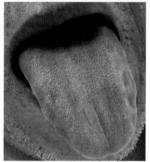

图 3.2.4.7a
Fig.3.2.4.7a

图 3.2.4.7b
Fig.3.2.4.7b

（八）肺胀 – 痰湿蕴肺证

4.8　Lung distention: syndrome of phlegm-dampness accumulating lung

患者刘某，男，57 岁，间断咳嗽、喘息 10 余年，加重 15 天，于 2016 年 11 月 27 日就诊。

Patient Liu, male, 57 years old, had been suffering from intermittent cough and dyspnea for more than 10 years. The symptoms aggravated 15 days ago, so he came to visit the doctor on November 27, 2016.

患者咳嗽、喘息 10 余年，间断中西药物治疗，具体不详。刻诊：慢性病容，呼吸急促，咳嗽，咳白色黏痰，不易咯出，不得平卧，胸闷喘息，活动后加重，纳食尚可，夜寐差，大便偏稀，小便平。颈静脉充盈，桶状胸，双肺叩之过清音，听诊双下肺细湿性啰音，舌质暗红，苔白腻（图 3.2.4.8a），脉弦滑。

The patient had cough and wheezing for more than 10 years and was intermittently treated with Chinese and Western medicine. Present symptoms: chronic disease appearance, tachypnea, cough with difficult expectoration of sticky white phlegm, inability to lie flat, chest distress and dyspnea that aggravated with movement, normal appetite, poor sleep, loose stool, normal urine, fullness of jugular vein, barrel chest, hyperresonance in the lungs, and wet rales in the lower lungs, dark red tongue with white greasy fur (Fig.3.2.4.8a), and wiry slippery pulse.

中医诊断：肺胀。

TCM diagnosis: lung distention.

辨证：痰湿阻肺，气机不畅证。

Syndrome differentiation: phlegm-dampness obstructing lung, inhibition of qi movement.

治疗：燥湿化痰，理气调中。

Treatment: drying dampness and resolving phlegm, regulating qi and the middle energizer.

处方：二陈汤加减：炒白术 15g，茯苓 15g，陈皮 10g，法半夏 10g，杏仁 10g，厚朴 10g，枳壳 10g，海浮石 15g，炙麻黄 6g，黄芩 10g，麦芽 15g，冬瓜子 15g，丹参 15g，郁金 10g，甘草 5g。7 剂，日 1 剂，水煎服。

Prescription: modified *Erchen* Decoction.

Chaobaizhu 15g, fuling 15g, chenpi 10g, fabanxia 10g, xingren 10g, houpo 10g, zhike 10g, haifushi 15g, zhimahuang 6g, huanglin 10g, maiya 15g, dongguazi 15g, danshen 15g, yujin 10g, gancao 5g.

Seven doses and one dose a day, decoction.

证候分析：久病咳喘，耗伤脾肺，脾气不足，津液运行疏布失职而生痰湿，痰湿贮存于肺，肺气上逆则咳嗽，咳白色黏痰，胸闷喘息；脾肺气虚，则活动后胸闷喘息加重；湿阻气滞而成血瘀，可见舌质暗红；苔白腻，脉弦滑为痰湿内蕴之象。

Syndrome analysis: long-term cough and asthma damages the spleen and lung. Insufficiency of spleen qi and abnormal spreading of fluid produces phlegm-dampness that is stored in the lung. Lung qi ascending counterflow causes cough, expectoration of sticky white phlegm, chest distress, and dyspnea. Qi deficiency of lung and spleen explains chest distress and dyspnea that aggravated with movement. Dampness obstruction and qi stagnation produces blood stasis, therefore, there appears dark red tongue. White greasy tongue fur and wiry slippery pulse suggest internal accumulation of phlegm-dampness.

2016年12月5日二诊：精神可，咳嗽咳痰症状减轻，可以平卧，呼吸平稳，舌质淡红，苔薄白（图3.2.4.8b），脉滑。维持原方治疗。

Second visit on December 5, 2016: cough and expectoration were alleviated, and the patient had normal spirit, ability to lie flat, stable respiration, light red tongue with thin white fur (Fig.3.2.4.8b), and slippery pulse. The previous prescription was used for treatment.

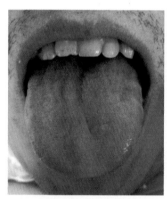 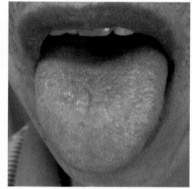

图 3.2.4.8a
Fig.3.2.4.8a

图 3.2.4.8b
Fig.3.2.4.8b

（九）乳蛾 – 肺经风热证

4.9 Tonsillitis: syndrome of wind-heat in lung meridian

患者王某，男，41岁，咽痛10天伴发热3天，于2017年4月30日就诊。

Patient Wang, male, 41 years old, had been suffering from sore throat for 10 days and a fever for 3 days, so he came to visit the doctor on April 30, 2017.

患者10天前熬夜后咽喉肿痛，口服药物而症状不减，3天前咽痛症状加重，伴高热，遂来就诊。刻诊：发热，伴寒战，咽痛，咽干，咳嗽，以干咳为主，偶咳少许白痰，前额及两侧头痛，口干欲饮，口苦，无胸痛胸闷，无呕吐，左下腹疼痛不适，食纳尚可，大便溏，小便平，舌质红，苔薄黄（图 3.2.4.9a），脉滑数。

The patient had sore throat after staying up late 10 days ago. After oral medication, the symptom wasn't relieved. The sore throat aggravated 3 days ago, accompanied by high fever, therefore, he came to see the doctor. Present symptoms: fever with chills, dry and sore throat, cough (mainly dry cough) with occasional scanty white phlegm, headache in the forehead and both sides, dry mouth with desire to drink, bitter taste in the mouth, no chest pain and distress, no vomiting, pain in the left lower abdomen, normal appetite, loose stool, normal urine, red tongue with thin yellow fur (Fig.3.2.4.9a), and rapid slippery pulse.

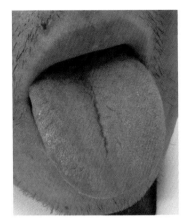

图 3.2.4.9
Fig.3.2.4.9

西医诊断：急性化脓性扁桃体炎。

Western medicine diagnosis: acute suppurative tonsillitis.

中医诊断：乳蛾。

TCM diagnosis: tonsillitis.

辨证：肺经风热，闭阻肺窍证。

Syndrome differentiation: wind-heat obstructing lung.

治疗：疏风清热，宣肺止咳。

Treatment: dispersing wind and clearing heat, ventilating lung and relieving cough.

处方：桑菊饮加减：桑叶 10g，菊花 10g，桔梗 10g，杏仁 10g，连翘 12g，黄芩 10g，北沙参 15g，芦根 12g，浙贝母 6g，薄荷 6g（后下），生甘草 5g。5 剂，日 1 剂，水煎服。

Prescription: modified *Sangju* Decoction.

Sangye 10g, juhua 10g, jiegeng 10g, xingren 10g, lianqiao 12g, huangqin 10g, beishashen 15g, lugen 12g, zhebeimu 6g, bohe 6g (decocted later), shenggancao 5g.

Five doses and one dose a day, decoction.

证候分析：风热之邪侵袭肺系，伤津耗液，肺失宣降，出现干咳少痰；热邪上灼，现咽痛、口干；舌质红，苔薄黄，脉滑数，为风热内侵肺系之明证。

Syndrome analysis: pathogenic wind-heat invading lung causes body fluid consumption and dysfunction of the lung to disperse and descend, so dry cough with scanty phlegm happen. Pathogenic heat burning upward causes sore throat and dry mouth. Red tongue with thin yellow fur and slippery rapid pulse are manifestations of internal invasion of wind-heat in the lung.

2017 年 5 月 5 日：患者来电告知，诸症痊愈。嘱清淡饮食，多喝开水。

May 5, 2017: the patient phoned that all the symptoms were removed. And he was asked to maintain light diet and drink plenty of boiled water.

（十）肺痈 – 痰热蕴肺证

4.10　Lung abscess: syndrome of phlegm-heat accumulating lung

患者刘某，男，64 岁，咳嗽、咯痰 10 余年加重 1 月，于 2016 年 11 月 12 日就诊。

Patient Liu, male, 64 years old, had cough and expectoration for more than 10 years. The symptoms aggravated for one month, so he came to visit the doctor on November 12, 2016.

患者支气管扩张 10 余年，时有咳嗽咯浓痰，近 1 月来因劳累而致咳嗽、咳痰症状加重，于某医院行抗生素输液治疗，症状不减，遂来就诊。刻诊：咳嗽时作，咯痰日数口至十数口，咳甚时痰中带血、胸闷、气憋，时有汗出，口干口渴，纳差，寐差，大便偏干，小便平，舌质暗，苔黄腻（图 3.2.4.10a），脉滑数。

The patient had bronchiectasis for more than 10 years, with occasional cough and expectoration of thick phlegm. The symptoms aggravated for one month due to fatigue, and an antibiotic infusion treatment in the hospital didn't work well, so he came to visit the doctor. Present symptoms: frequent cough with expectoration of several mouthful or dozens of mouthful phlegm daily, bloody phlegm when cough was severe, chest oppression, depression of qi, occasional sweating, dry mouth and thirst, poor appetite and sleep, slightly dry stool, normal urine, dark tongue with yellow greasy fur (Fig.3.2.4.10a), and slippery rapid pulse.

西医诊断：肺脓疡。

Western medicine diagnosis: lung abscess.

中医诊断：肺痈。

TCM diagnosis: lung abscess.

辨证：痰热蕴肺，肺失宣肃证。

Syndrome differentiation: phlegm-heat accumulating lung, failure of lung to depurate and descend.

治疗：清热解毒，肃肺化痰。

Treatment: clearing heat and removing toxin, descending qi and resolving phlegm.

处方：千金苇茎汤加减：炒薏苡仁 20g，桃仁 10g，冬瓜子 15g，全瓜蒌 15g，茯苓 15g，百部 10g，蛤蚧 10g，赤芍 12g，白豆蔻 15g。7 剂，日 1 剂，水煎服。

Prescription: modified *Qianjin Weijing* Decoction.

Chaoyiyiren 20g, taoren 10g, dongguazi 15g, quangualou 15g, fuling 15g, baibu 10g, gejie 10g, chishao 12g, baidoukou 15g.

Seven doses and one dose a day, decoction.

证候分析：邪热壅肺，日久蕴酿成痈，肺失宣降，出现胸闷气憋，咳嗽咯痰；邪热熏蒸肺络，出现痰中带血；邪热蒸迫津液，故汗出；舌质暗，苔黄腻，脉滑数，为痰热蕴结在肺之象。

Syndrome analysis: long-term pathogenic heat accumulatinglunggenerates lung carbuncle. Dysfunction of the lung in dispersing and descending causes chest oppression, depression of qi, cough and expectoration. Pathogenic heat damaging the lung collaterals causes blood-stained phlegm. Pathogenic heat steaming body fluid outward causes sweating. Dark red tongue with yellow greasy fur and slippery rapid pulse indicate phlegm-heat accumulating lung.

2016 年 11 月 19 日二诊：咳嗽咳痰明显减轻，痰量明显减少，痰中带血，口干，无胸闷、气憋，大小便正常，舌淡红，苔薄黄（图 3.2.4.10b），脉滑。原方加蒲黄炭 12g、北沙参 30g，7 剂，巩固治疗。

Second visit on November 19, 2016: the syndromes of cough and expectoration obviously alleviated, with obvious decrease of phlegm amount. But the patient still had bloody phlegm, dry mouth, no chest oppression and depression of qi, normal stool and urine, light red tongue with thin yellow fur (Fig.3.2.4.10b), and slippery pulse. Seven doses of the previous prescription were used to consolidate the effect, with the addition of puhuangtan 12g and beishashen 30g.

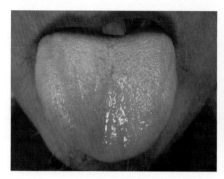 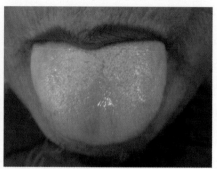

图 3.2.4.10a

Fig.3.2.4.10a

图 3.2.4.10b

Fig.3.2.4.10b

（十一）失音 – 肺燥津伤证

4.11　Aphonia: syndrome of lung dryness damaging fluid

患者汪某，女，26 岁，声音嘶哑 2 月，于 2015 年 11 月 23 日就诊。

Patient Wang, female, 26 years old, had been suffering from a hoarseness for more than 2 months, so she visited the doctor on November 23, 2015.

患者是一名教师，连续上课导致声音嘶哑，曾用中药泡茶饮，症状有所好转，但课堂声音稍大即音哑，为求规范化治疗而就诊。刻诊：声音嘶哑，口燥咽干，周身乏力，偶有咳嗽，干咳少痰，纳食尚可，大便偏干，小便少，舌质红，少苔（图 3.2.4.11a），脉细数。

The patient is a teacher and continuous lessons caused her hoarse voice. She once drank Chinese herbal tea, with the symptom improved. But her voice became hoarse with louder voice in class. Therefore she came to visit the doctor for systematic treatment. Present symptoms: hoarse voice, dry mouth, fatigue, occasional dry cough with scanty phlegm, normal appetite, slightly dry stool, scanty urine, red tongue with little fur (Fig.3.2.4.11a), and thready rapid pulse.

中医诊断：失音。

TCM diagnosis: aphonia.

辨证：肺燥津伤证。

Syndrome differentiation: lung dryness damaging fluid.

治疗：清燥救肺，生津利咽。

Treatment: clearing dryness and moistening lung, promoting fluid production and disinhibiting throat.

处方：清燥润肺汤加减：北沙参 30g，麦冬 15g，枇杷叶 10g，杏仁 10g，木蝴蝶 15g，诃子 10g，石斛 10g，火麻仁 15g，马勃 10g，川贝母 6g。7 剂，日 1 剂，水煎服。

Prescription: modified *Qingzao Runfei* Decoction.

Beishashen 30g, maidong 15g, pipaye 10g, xingren 10g, muhudie 15g, hezi 10g, shihu 10g, huomaren 15g, mabo 10g, chuanbeimu 6g.

Seven doses and one dose a day, decoction.

证候分析：久语耗气伤阴，肺阴不足，咽喉失润，则音哑、喉燥、口干；肺阴不足，虚火内灼，肺失清肃，气逆于上，故干咳少痰；舌红，苔薄少，脉细数，为阴虚内热之象。

Syndrome analysis: excessive talking damages qi and yin. Lung yin insufficiency cannot moisten the throat, hoarse voice, dry mouth and throat appear. Lung yin insufficiency and internal scorching of deficiency fire causes failure of lung to depurate and descend as well as adverse rising of qi, so dry cough with scanty phlegm occurs. Red tongue with thin little fur and thready rapid pulse suggest yin deficiency with internal heat.

2015 年 11 月 30 日二诊：患者精神佳，语言清晰无嘶哑，无口干、咽干，二便可，舌淡红、苔薄（图 3.2.4.11b），脉细。原方 5 剂巩固治疗。嘱常以麦冬、沙参、胖大海泡水喝，多饮开水，注意用嗓。

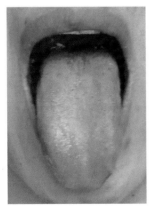 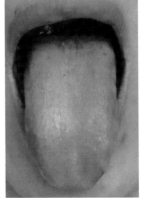

图 3.2.4.11a　　　　　　　图 3.2.4.11b
Fig.3.2.4.11a　　　　　　　Fig.3.2.4.11b

Second visit on November 30, 2015: the patient had good spirit, clear speech without hoarse voice, no dry mouth or throat, normal stool and urine, light red tongue with thin fur (Fig.3.2.4.11b), and thready pulse. Five doses of the previous prescription were used to consolidate the efficacy. And she was advised to drink more boiled water and medicated tea made from maidong, shashen and pangdahai, and pay more attention to healthy use of the voice.

（十二）咯血 – 肝火犯肺证

4.12 Hemoptysis: syndrome of liver fire invading lung

患者黄某，女，70 岁，咳嗽咳痰 10 天加重 1 天，于 2017 年 4 月 24 日就诊。

Patient Huang, female, 70 years old, had been suffering from cough and expectoration for 10 days, and the symptoms aggravated for one day, so she came to visit the doctor on April 24, 2017.

患者 10 天前因情志不舒后出现剧烈咳嗽，咳甚腹痛，咳黄痰，用药物治疗（具体用药不详），上述症状减轻，但仍间断咳嗽。1 天前夜间无明显诱因出现咯血，色鲜红，量多，不能自行缓解，今为求进一步诊治而来就诊。刻诊：精神抑郁，咯血，痰中带血、色鲜红，咳嗽咳痰，黏痰而黄，量少，易咯出，头痛头晕，近段时间身体消瘦约 5kg，无盗汗，无恶寒发热，无口干口苦，无鼻塞流涕，无胸痛，纳食可，夜寐差，二便调。舌质紫暗、苔黄（图 3.2.4.12a），脉弦数。

The patient suffered from severe cough 10 days ago due to emotional discomfort, accompanied with abdominal pain and expectoration of yellow phlegm. The above symptoms were relieved by medication (specific medicines were unknown), but the intermittent cough still persisted. Without obvious inducement, she had hemoptysis at nighttime with bright red color and large amount one day ago. And the hemoptysis couldn't be self-alleviated, so she came to see the doctor for further treatment. Present symptoms: mental depression, hemoptysis, bloody phlegm with bright red color, cough and easy expectoration of scanty yellow and sticky phlegm, headache and dizziness, 5 kg of lose weight recently, no night sweating, no aversion to cold or fever, no dry mouth or bitter taste in the mouth, no nasal congestion or running nose, no chest pain, normal appetite, poor sleep, normal urine and stool, purple dark tongue with yellow fur (Fig.3.2.4.12a), and wiry rapid pulse.

既往史：睡眠障碍史 40 余年；10 年前因阑尾炎行阑尾切除术；腰椎间盘突出 3 年，未系统治疗。否认高血压、糖尿病、心脏病史，否认肝炎、结核病史，无重大外伤史，无输血史，预防接种史随当地进行。

Past medical history: somnipathy for more than 40 years; appendectomy for more than 10 years because of appendicitis; prolapse of lumbar intervertebral disc for 3 years without systematic treatment; denial history of hypertension, diabetes, heart disease, hepatitis, tuberculosis, severe trauma, and blood transfusion; and local-requirement-followed vaccination history.

西医诊断：咯血（原因待查）。

Western medicine diagnosis: hemoptysis (its cause was to be examined).

中医诊断：咯血。

TCM diagnosis: hemoptysis.

辨证：肝火犯肺，肺失宣肃证。

Syndrome differentiation: liver fire invading lung, failure of lung to disperse and descend.

治疗：清热平肝，化痰止咳。

Treatment: clearing heat and pacifying liver, resolving phlegm and relieving cough.

处方：化肝煎加减：青皮 10g，陈皮 10g，栀子 15g，牡丹皮 10g，泽泻 10g，浙贝母 10g，全瓜蒌 15g，白芷 10g，白芍 15g，鱼腥草 15g，血余炭 15g，炒蒲黄 15g，生地炭 15g，生姜 3 片。7 剂，日 1 剂，水煎服。

Prescription: modified *Huagan* Decoction.

Qingpi 10g, chenpi 10g, zhizi 15g, mudanpi 10g, zexie 10g, zhebeimu 10g, quangualou 15g, baizhi 10g, baishao 15g, yuxingcao 15g, xueyutan 15g, chaopuhuang 15g, shengditan 15g, shengjiang 3 pieces.

Seven doses and one dose a day, decoction.

证候分析：患者平素精神抑郁，日久化火，肝火上逆侵肺，出现咳嗽、咳痰而黄；火热之邪灼伤肺络，而见咳血；舌质紫暗、苔黄主热，加之脉弦数，为肝火犯肺之征。

Syndrome analysis: long-term mental depression transforming into fire and up-flaming of liver fire invading lung cause cough and expectoration of yellow phlegm. Pathogenic fire-heat scorches the lung collaterals, so hemoptysis appears. Dark purple tongue with yellow fur and wiry rapid pulse indicate liver fire invading lung, of which yellow fur also suggests heat syndrome.

2017 年 5 月 2 日二诊：患者精神佳，无咳嗽、咯血，无头痛头晕，夜寐差，入睡困难，易于惊醒，舌质淡紫，苔薄黄（图 3.2.4.12b），脉弦。血常规示：红细胞（＋）。原方加夜交藤 30g、合欢皮 20g、珍珠母 30g，7 剂。逍遥丸调理善后。

Second visit on May 2, 2017: the patient had good spirit, no cough or hemoptysis, no headache or dizziness, difficult sleeping with easy wake-up, light purple tongue with thin yellow fur (Fig.3.2.4.12b), and wiry pulse. Blood routine test: RBC (+). Seven doses of the previous prescription were used for treatment, with the addition of yejiaoteng 30g, hehuanpi 20g, and zhenzhumu 30g. After medication, *Xiaoyao* Pill was used for rehabilitation.

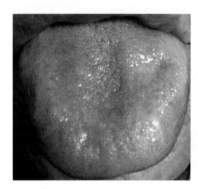 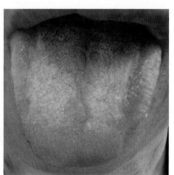

图 3.2.4.12a
Fig.3.2.4.12a

图 3.2.4.12b
Fig.3.2.4.12b

五、肾系病证

5. Kidney system syndrome

（一）水肿 – 脾肾阳虚证

5.1　Edema: syndrome of yang deficiency of spleen and kidney

患者申某，女，43 岁，颜面肢体浮肿 7 天，于 2012 年 5 月 5 日就诊。

Patient Shen, female, 43 years old, had been suffering from facial edema for 7 days. So she came to see the doctor on May 5, 2012.

患者 3 年前患急性肾炎，经某医院治疗，尿蛋白消失后出院。之后因感冒、劳累等原因，病情常反复，肢体水肿时起时消，缠绵难愈。7 天前因受风寒而出现面浮肢肿，遂来就诊。刻诊：神疲乏力，颜面肢体浮肿，下肢脚踝肿甚，腰背酸冷，小便短少，大便溏泻，舌质淡，苔白而滑（图 3.2.5.1a），脉沉无力。尿常规示：蛋白质（+++），管型（0 ～ ++），红细胞（0 ～ ++）。血常规示：红细胞 3.8×10^{12}/L，血红蛋白

97g/L，白细胞 7.34 × 10^9/L。

Three years ago, the patient suffered with acute nephritis and discharged from the hospital after the disappearance of urine protein. Then, the disease was often repeated because of cold, fatigue and other factors, with the persistent and intermittent limb edema. The patient had facial and limb edema 7 days ago because of cold attack, so she came to see the doctor. Present symptoms: fatigue, facial and limb edema, especially the ankles, aching cold in the back and waist, scanty urine, loose stool, pale tongue with white slippery fur (Fig.3.2.5.1a), and deep powerless pulse. Routine urine test: protein (+++), urinary cast (0-++), RBC (0-++). Blood routine test: RBC 3.8 × 10^{12}/L, Hb 97g/L, WBC 7.34 × 10^9/L.

西医诊断：急性肾小球肾炎。

Western medicine diagnosis: acute glomerulonephritis.

中医诊断：水肿。

TCM diagnosis: edema.

辨证：脾肾阳虚，气不化水证。

Syndrome differentiation: yang deficiency of spleen and kidney and qi failing to transform water.

治疗：温阳健脾，利水消肿。

Treatment: warming yang and invigorating spleen, draining water to alleviate edema.

处方：苓桂术甘汤加减：茯苓皮 15g，猪苓 15g，桂枝 10g，炒白术 15g，制附子 6g（先煎），车前子 15g（包煎），炒薏苡仁 20g，橘络 10g，益母草 15g，大腹皮 10g，生姜 3 片，炙甘草 5g。7 剂，日 1 剂，水煎服。

Prescription: modified *Lingui Zhugan* Decoction.

Fulingpi 15g, zhuling 15g, guizhi 10g, chaobaizhu 15g, zhifuzi 6g (decocted first), cheqianzi 15g (wrap-boiling), chaoyiyiren 20g, juluo 10g, yimucao 15g, dafupi 10g, shengjiang 3 pieces, zhigancao 5g.

Seven doses and one dose a day, decoction.

证候分析：脾肾阳虚，气化失职，水液不循常道，则小便短少、大便稀溏；水液外溢肌肤，出现肢体、颜面水肿；阳虚失却温煦，则腰背酸冷；舌质淡，苔白而滑，脉沉无力，乃脾肾阳虚，温润、鼓动无力所致。

Syndrome analysis: yang deficiency of spleen and kidney and dysfunction of qi transformation causes the liquid failing to follow the ordinary course, scanty urine and stool loose. Water-fluid overflowing outward into the skin causes facial and limb edema. Yang deficiency induces dysfunction of warming, so the patient had aching cold in the back and waist. Pale tongue with white slippery fur and deep powerless pulse is caused by yang deficiency of spleen and kidney that fails to fulfill its warming, moistening and propelling functions.

2012 年 5 月 13 日二诊：颜面水肿消失，双下肢脚踝水肿明显减轻，小便量多，舌淡，苔白（图 3.2.5.1b），脉沉。证情稳定，嘱服金匮肾气丸巩固疗效。

Second visit on May 13, 2012: facial edema was disappeared and the edema of the ankles was reduced significantly. The patient had profuse urine, pale tongue with white fur (Fig.3.2.5.1b), and deep pulse. After the condition stabilized, *Jingui Shenqi* Pill was prescribed to consolidate curative effect.

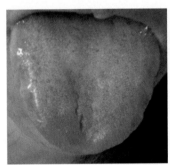 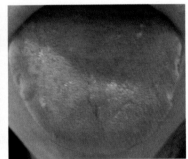

图 3.2.5.1a　　　　　　　　　图 3.2.5.1b
Fig.3.2.5.1a　　　　　　　　　Fig.3.2.5.1b

（二）水肿 – 脾肾阳虚证

5.2　Edema: syndrome of yang deficiency of spleen and kidney

患者王某，女，43 岁，双下肢浮肿 2 年加重 1 月，于 2015 年 4 月 10 日就诊。

Patient Wang, female, 43 years old, had been suffering from edema in lower limbs for 2 years and the symptom aggravated for one month, so she came to see the doctor on April 10, 2015.

患者 2 年前无明显诱因出现双下肢浮肿，某医院诊断为肾小球肾炎，间断服双氢克尿噻、安体舒通治疗，症状有所缓解。近 1 月来患者因劳累而双下肢浮肿增重，遂来就诊。刻诊：精神差，疲乏无力，面色㿠白虚浮，双下肢浮肿，按之凹陷不起，两腿沉重无力，自汗、短气，带下量多，已绝经，小便量少，大便偏溏，舌淡伴齿痕，苔白腻（图 3.2.5.2a），脉弱。尿常规：蛋白质（++），管型（+），红细胞（3～5个）。血常规：血红蛋白 100g/L。肾功能：尿素氮（－），肌酐（－）。

The patient had edema in lower limbs with no obvious inducement 2 years ago and she was diagnosed as glomerulonephritis. Then, she took hydrochlorothiazide and spironolactone intermittently for treatment, with the symptoms alleviated. In recent one month, the edema in lower limbs aggravated due to fatigue, so she came to see the doctor. Present symptoms: poor spirit, fatigue and lassitude, bright white complexion, puffy face, pitting edema in lower limbs, heaviness and weakness in legs, spontaneous sweating, shortness of breath, profuse leucorrhea, menopause, scanty urine, loose stool, pale teeth-marked tongue with white greasy fur (Fig.3.2.5.2a), and weak pulse. Routine urine test: protein (++), urinary cast (+), RBC (3-5). Blood routine test: Hb 100g/L. Renal function: BUN (-), Scr (-).

西医诊断：慢性肾小球肾炎。

Western medicine diagnosis: chronic glomerulonephritis.

中医诊断：水肿。

TCM diagnosis: edema.

辨证：脾肾阳虚，气化不利证。

Syndrome differentiation: yang deficiency of spleen and kidney, and disturbance of qi transformation.

治疗：健脾补肾，温阳利水。

Treatment: invigorating spleen and tonifying kidney, warming yang and draining water.

处方：防己黄芪汤加减：黄芪 30g，党参 15g，防己 15g，炒白术 15g，茯苓 15g，大腹皮 15g，泽泻 10g，鸡内金 10g，生姜 3 片，木瓜 10g，大枣 3 枚。7 剂，日 1 剂，水煎服。

Prescription: modified *Fangji Huangqi* Decoction.

Huangqi 30g, dangshen 15g, fangji 15g, chaobaizhu 15g, fuling 15g, dafupi 15g, zexie 10g, jineijin 10g, shengjiang 3 pieces, mugua 10g, dazao 3 pieces.

Seven doses and one dose a day, decoction.

证候分析：脾肾阳虚，气化不利，水液不循常道，泛溢肌肤，而见面白虚浮、双下肢浮肿；阳虚不固，则自汗、女子带下量多；阳虚温煦、气化失职，见小便量少、大便溏泻；舌淡伴齿痕，苔白腻，脉弱，为脾肾阳虚之象。

Syndrome analysis: yang deficiency of spleen and kidney and disturbance of qi transformation causes water-fluid failing to follow the ordinary course and overflowing into the skin, there appear the symptoms such as pale complexion, puffy face, and edema in lower limbs. Yang deficiency causes dysfunction of kidney to secure, so the symptoms such as spontaneous sweating and profuse leucorrhea appear. Yang deficiency induces dysfunction of warming and qi transformation, so the symptoms of scanty urine and loose stool appear. Pale teeth-marked tongue with white greasy fur and weak pulse are the manifestations of yang deficiency of spleen and kidney.

2015 年 4 月 17 日二诊：精神较前好转，双下肢浮肿减轻，舌淡，苔白（图 3.2.5.2b），脉沉。继服前方 14 剂后，诸症悉除。

Second visit on April 17, 2015: the spirit was better than before and edema in lower limbs was relieved. The patient had pale tongue with white fur (Fig.3.2.5.2b), and deep pulse. Fourteen doses of the original prescription were used for treatment. After medication, all the symptoms were disappeared.

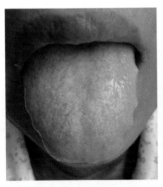 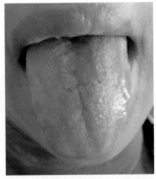

图 3.2.5.2a
Fig.3.2.5.2a

图 3.2.5.2b
Fig.3.2.5.2b

（三）水肿 – 脾肾气虚证

5.3　Edema: syndrome of qi deficiency of spleen and kidney

患者陈某，男，45 岁，发现血压高、肾功能异常 3 年，双下肢浮肿 1 月，于 2015 年 11 月 7 日就诊。

Patient Chen, male, 45 years old, was diagnosed as high blood pressure and abnormal renal function 3 years ago. He suffered from edema in lower limbs one month ago and came to see the doctor on November 7, 2015.

患者 3 年前因血压高、肾功能异常于某医院诊断为"高血压病、慢性肾衰竭",间断服用降压、降肌酐、降蛋白尿药物治疗,效果不佳,肌酐逐渐上升。近 1 月来患者双下肢浮肿明显,遂来就诊。刻诊:面色㿠白,精神差,双眼睑浮肿,头晕,心慌,纳差,口淡不渴,无恶心、呕吐,双下肢凹陷性水肿,腰膝酸软,寐差,大便溏,小便量少,舌淡嫩伴齿痕瘀点,苔薄白水滑(图 3.2.5.3a),脉沉细。辅助检查:肌酐 900 μmol/L。

The patient had high blood pressure and abnormal renal function 3 years ago, and he was diagnosed as hypertension and chronic renal failure. Intermittent administration of antihypertensive, creatinine-reducing and proteinuria-reducing drugs has poor results and creatinine gradually increases. In recent one month, edema in lower limbs was obvious and he came to see the doctor. Present symptoms: bright white complexion, poor spirit, edema in the eyelids, dizziness, flusteredness, poor appetite, tastelessness in the mouth without thirst, no nausea and vomiting, pitting edema in lower limbs, soreness and weakness of the waist and knees, poor sleep, loose stool, scanty urine, pale tender tongue with teeth marks, ecchymosis, and thin white and slippery fur (Fig.3.2.5.3a), and deep thready pulse. Auxiliary examination: Scr 900 μmol/L.

西医诊断:慢性肾脏病 5 期;高血压性肾病。

Western medicine diagnosis: chronic renal disease (the fifth phase) ; hypertensive nephropathy.

中医诊断:水肿。

TCM diagnosis: edema.

辨证:脾肾气虚证。

Syndrome differentiation: qi deficiency of spleen and kidney.

治疗:健脾益肾,利水消肿。

Treatment: invigorating spleen and replenishing kidney, and draining water to alleviate edema.

处方:六君子汤加减:黄芪 15g,党参 15g,炒白术 15g,茯苓 20g,猪苓 15g,白扁豆 15g,炒莱菔子 15g,龙眼肉 10g,酸枣仁 20g,牛膝 20g,杜仲 15g,桑寄生 20g,淫羊藿 10g,砂仁 5g(后下),甘草 5g。7 剂,日 1 剂,水煎服。

Prescription: modified *Liujunzi* Decoction.

Huangqi 15g, dangshen 15g, chaobaizhu 15g, fuling 20g, zhuling 15g, baibiandou 15g, chaolaifuzi 15g, longyanrou 10g, suanzaoren 20g, niuxi 20g, duzhong 15g, sangjisheng 20g, yinyanghuo 10g, sharen 5g（decocted later), gancao 5g.

Seven doses and one dose a day, decoction.

证候分析：脾肾气虚，气化无权，致水湿内聚，不循常道，泛溢肌肤，而见水肿；水气凌心射肺，可致胸闷、气促等症；脾虚，气血生化不足，心神失养，则心慌、寐差；气血不足，不能上荣清窍，则头晕；脾虚，运化无力，则纳差、口淡不渴；肾虚，腰府失养，则腰膝酸软；肾虚，膀胱开阖失职，可见尿少或无尿；舌淡紫伴齿痕，苔薄白水滑，为脾肾气虚，无力鼓动至血瘀、水停之征象。

Syndrome analysis: qi deficiency of spleen and kidney and dysfunction of qi transformation causes internal accumulation of water-dampness and its overflowing into the skin, so edema appears. Retention of fluid attacks heart and lung, so the symptoms such as chest distress and dyspnea appear. Spleen deficiency induces insufficient generation and transformation of qi and blood and insufficient nourishment of heart spirit, so flusteredness and poor sleep appear. The insufficiency of qi and blood failing to nourish the lucid orifices leads to dizziness. Spleen deficiency with the dysfunction of transformation and transportation explains poor appetite and tastelessness in the mouth without thirst. Kidney deficiency fails to nourish the waist, so soreness and weakness of the waist and knees appears. Kidney deficiency with dysfunction of bladder in opening and closing causes scanty urine or anuria. Light purple tongue with teeth mark and thin white and slippery fur are the signs of qi deficiency of spleen and kidney which causes blood stasis and water retention.

2015 年 11 月 14 日二诊：患者精神可，面色萎黄，双眼睑无浮肿，无头晕心慌，双下肢水肿减轻，腰膝酸软，大小便正常，舌淡红，苔薄白（图 3.2.5.3b），脉沉。原方加巴戟天 15g、怀牛膝 20g，7 剂。

Second visit on November 14, 2015: the patient had normal spirit, sallow complexion, no edema in the eyelids, no dizziness and flusteredness, alleviated edema in lower limbs, soreness and weakness of the waist and knees, normal stool and urine, light red tongue with thin white fur (Fig.3.2.5.3b), and deep pulse. Seven doses of the original prescription were used to consolidate the effect, with the addition of bajitian 15g and huainiuxi 20g.

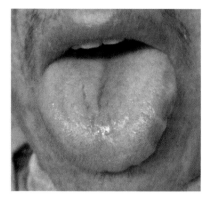

图 3.2.5.3a

Fig.3.2.5.3a

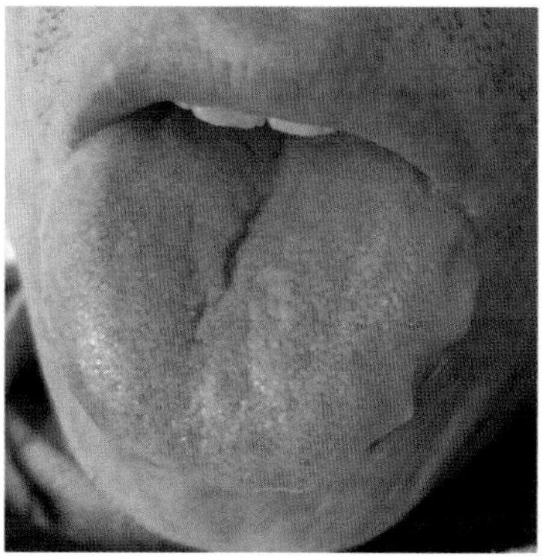

图 3.2.5.3b

Fig.3.2.5.3b

（四）水肿 – 脾肾气虚证

5.4　Edema: syndrome of spleen-kidney qi deficiency

患者吴某，男，74 岁，肾功能差多年，颜面及双下肢浮肿 1 月，于 2014 年 6 月 16 日就诊。

Patient Wu, male, 74 years old, had been suffering from poor renal function for many years, and had edema in face and lower limbs for one month, so he came to see the doctor on June 16, 2014.

刻诊：精神可，颜面及双下肢浮肿伴头晕，乏力，恶心呕吐，发热，无咳嗽、咯痰，无关节疼痛，纳差，眠可，大便正常，夜尿 3～4 次，24 小时尿量约 1000mL，舌质淡，苔白腻（图 3.2.5.4a），脉沉弱。肾功能：尿素氮 30.7mmol/L，肌酐 989.4μmol/L，尿酸 454μmol/L。

Present symptoms: normal spirit, edema in the face and lower limbs, accompanied with dizziness, fatigue, nausea, vomiting, fever, no cough and expectoration, no joint pain, poor appetite, normal sleep, normal stool, enuresis nocturna 3-4 times, 1000mL of urine in 24 hours, pale tongue with white greasy fur (Fig.3.2.5.4a), and deep weak pulse. Renal function: BUN 30.7mmol/L, Scr 989.4μmol/L, UA 454μmol/L.

西医诊断：慢性肾脏病 5 期（慢性肾病综合征）。

Western medicine diagnosis: chronic kidney disease (the fifth phase) (chronic nephritis syndrome).

中医诊断：水肿。

TCM diagnosis: edema.

辨证：脾肾不足，运化失职证。

Syndrome differentiation: deficiency of spleen and kidney, dysfunction of transportation and transformation.

治疗：补肾健脾，利水消肿。

Treatment: tonifying kidney and invigorating spleen, draining water to alleviate edema.

处方：四君子汤合六味地黄汤加减：黄芪 15g，党参 15g，炒白术 15g，法半夏 10g，生地黄 12g，车前子 10g，泽兰 10g，蝉蜕 8g，山茱萸 15g，山药 15g，茯苓 15g，泽泻 10g，徐长卿 15g，白花蛇舌草 15g，芡实 10g，丁香 10g，柿蒂 10g。7 剂，日 1 剂，水煎服。

Prescription: modified *Sijunzi* Decoction together with *Liuwei Dihuang* Decoction.

Huangqi 15g, dangshen 15g, chaobaizhu 15g, fabanxia 10g, shengdihuang 12g, cheqianzi 10g, zelan 10g, chantui 8g, shanzhuyu 15g, shanyao 15g, fuling 15g, zexie 10g, xuchangqing 15g, baihuasheshecao 15g, qianshi 10g, dingxiang 10g, shidi 10g.

Seven doses and one dose a day, decoction.

证候分析：脾肾气虚，气化无权，土不制水，可有水肿出现；脾气不足，运化功能欠佳可见恶心、呕吐、全身乏力；脾不升清精微，头部失养则头晕；舌淡，苔白腻，脉沉弱，为脾肾气虚之征。

Syndrome analysis: qi deficiency of spleen and kidney and dysfunction of qi transformation cause earth failing to control water, which leads to edema. Spleen qi deficiency and dysfunction of transportation and transformation lead to nausea, vomiting and fatigue. Spleen failing to ascend the clear causes insufficient nourishment of the head and dizziness. Pale tongue with white greasy fur and deep weak pulse are the manifestations of qi deficiency of spleen and kidney.

2014 年 6 月 23 日二诊：患者无颜面水肿，下肢水肿减轻，无呕吐、发热，纳可，舌淡红，苔白稍腻（图 3.2.5.4b），脉弱。原方 7 剂，继续治疗。

Second visit on June 23, 2014: the patient had no edema in the face, relieved edema in lower limb, no vomiting and fever, normal appetite, pale red tongue with white and slightly greasy fur (Fig.3.2.5.4b), and weak pulse. Seven doses of the original prescription were used for further treatment.

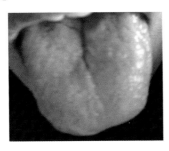
图 3.2.5.4a
Fig.3.2.5.4a

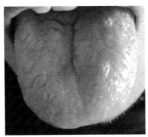
图 3.2.5.4b
Fig.3.2.5.4b

（五）水肿 – 肾气亏虚证
5.5　Edema: syndrome of kidney qi deficiency

患者刘某，男，41 岁，因发现肾功能异常 1 月余，于 2015 年 5 月 14 日就诊。

Patient Liu, male, 41 years old, had been suffering from renal dysfunction for one month, then he came to see the doctor on May 14, 2015.

患者 1 个月前因上楼感觉四肢乏力，两脚发软伴腹痛，于当地医院就诊，治疗后未见明显好转且出现颜面浮肿 7 天，遂来就诊。刻诊：全身乏力，颜面、肢体浮肿，脸有发热感，头右侧及后项轻度疼痛，腹痛伴恶心呕吐感，纳食差，腰膝酸软，小便量少，舌淡紫胖大伴齿痕，苔黄（图 3.2.5.5a），脉沉细弱。上腹部 B 超示：房间隔与左室后壁增厚，左房、左室增大，左室舒张功能减低，心包少量积液。肾功能：尿素氮 49.6mmol/L，肌酐 686.2μmol/L，尿酸 561μmol/L。

The patient felt weakness of four limbs accompanied with abdominal pain one month ago and was treated in local hospital without obvious efficacy. And after treatment, the patient had facial edema for 7 days, so he came to see the doctor. Present symptoms: fatigue, facial and limb edema, hot sensation in the face, mild pain in right and lateral side of the head, abdominal pain accompanied with nausea and vomiting, poor appetite, aching and weak waist and knees, scanty urine, pale purple enlarged tongue with teeth-marks and yellow fur (Fig.3.2.5.5a), and deep thready weak pulse. Upper abdomen B ultrasound: the interatrial septum and the posterior wall of left ventricle was thickened, the left atrium and left ventricle were enlarged, the left ventricular diastolic function was reduced, and a small amount of pericardial effusion. Renal function: BUN 49.6 mmol/L, Scr 686.2 μ mol/L, UA 561 μ mol/L.

西医诊断：慢性肾衰竭；慢性肾脏病 4 期。

Western medicine diagnosis: chronic renal failure, chronic kidney disease (the fourth phase).

中医诊断：水肿。

TCM diagnosis: edema.

辨证：肾气亏虚，气化不及证。

Syndrome differentiation: kidney qi deficiency and dysfunction of qi transformation.

治疗：健脾益肾，利水渗湿。

Treatment: invigorating spleen and replenishing kidney, draining water and percolating dampness.

处方：四君子汤合六味地黄汤加减：黄芪 20g，党参 15g，炒白术 15g，茯苓 20g，猪苓 10g，泽泻 10g，熟地黄 10g，山药 20g，山茱萸 10g，牡丹皮 10g，橘络 10g，牛膝 20g，杜仲 15g，甘草 3g。7 剂，日 1 剂，水煎服。

Prescription: modified *Sijunzi* Decoction together with *Liuwei Dihuang* Decoction.

Huangqi 20g, dangshen 15g, chaobaizhu 15g, fuling 20g, zhuling 10g, zexie 10g, shudihuang 10g, shanyao 20g, shanzhuyu 10g, mudanpi 10g, juluo 10g, niuxi 20g, duzhong 15g, gancao 3g.

Seven doses and one dose a day, decoction.

证候分析：患者脾肾气虚，气化无权，土不制水，可有颜面、肢体水肿出现；脾虚不运，则纳差；脾虚，水谷精微生成不足，不能充养肢体，则周身乏力；脾虚，中焦不运，升降失和，则恶心、呕吐；肾虚，腰府失养，则腰膝酸软；肾虚，膀胱气化失职，则小便量少；舌淡紫胖大伴齿痕、苔黄为水湿内盛，脉沉细弱为湿阻气机，脉道失充所致。

Syndrome analysis: qi deficiency of spleen and kidney and failure of qi transformation lead to facial and limb edema. Spleen qi deficiency with dysfunction in transportation causes poor appetite. Spleen qi deficiency cannot produce fine substances to nourish the body, which leads to general fatigue. Spleen deficiency causes the middle energizer failing to transportation and abnormal ascending and descending, so nausea and vomiting happens. Kidney deficiency and insufficient nourishment of the waist cause aching and weak waist and knees. Kidney deficiency and bladder's dysfunction in qi transformation causes scanty urine. Pale purple, enlarged tongue with teeth-marks and yellow fur suggests internal exuberance of dampness, and deep thready weak pulse is caused by dampness obstructing qi movement and insufficient blood of vessels.

2015 年 5 月 21 日二诊：患者精神可，所有症状均明显减轻，无腹痛，尿量增加，舌淡红苔黄（图 3.2.5.5b），脉沉。效不更方，守原方服用 10 剂，继续治疗。

Second visit on May 21, 2015: with all the symptoms alleviated obviously, the patient had normal spirit, no abdominal pain, increased urine, light red tongue with yellow fur (Fig. 3.2.5.5b), and deep pulse. 10 doses of the original prescription were still used for treatment.

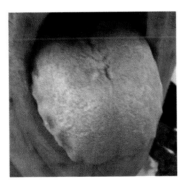 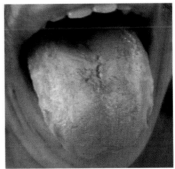

图 3.2.5.5a
Fig.3.2.5.5a

图 3.2.5.5b
Fig.3.2.5.5b

（六）淋证 – 肾阴不足，湿热下注证

5.6 Stranguria: syndrome of kidney yin deficiency and dampness-heat pouring downward

患者邹某，男，41 岁，小便不畅伴尿浊 5 年加重 1 月，于 2009 年 9 月 17 日就诊。

Patient Zou, male, 41 years old, had been suffering from unsmooth urination with urinary turbidity for 5 years and the symptoms aggravated one month ago, then he came to see the doctor on September 17, 2009.

患者患前列腺炎 5 年余，时常小便不畅，未系统治疗。近 1 月来，患者小便不畅伴有尿液浑浊，遂来就诊。刻诊：形体消瘦，面色晦暗，心烦少寐，口干欲饮，小便赤涩、疼痛不畅伴有白色浑浊物从尿中排出，大便时溏而不爽，舌质红，苔薄黄（图 3.2.5.6a），脉沉细。B 超示：前列腺增大，右肾盂可见泥沙样结石。

The patient had been suffering from prostatitis with unsmooth urination for more than 5 years and didn't receive systematic treatment. In the past one month, the patient had impeded urination with urinary turbidity, so he came to see the doctor. Present symptoms: emaciation, dark complexion, vexation and less sleep, thirsty with desire to drink, red unsmooth painful urination with white turbidity, unsmooth defecation with loose stool, red tongue with thin yellow fur (Fig.3.2.5.6a), and deep thin pulse. B-ultrasound: enlarged prostate and sediment-like stones in the right renal pelvis.

西医诊断：肾结石。

Western medicine diagnosis: renal calculus.

中医诊断：淋证。

TCM diagnosis: stranguria.

辨证：肾阴不足，湿热下注证。

Syndrome differentiation: kidney yin deficiency and dampness-heat pouring downward.

治疗：补肾阴，清湿热。

Treatment: nourishing kidney yin, and clearing dampness-heat.

处方：小蓟饮子加减：车前草 15g，北沙参 20g，丝瓜络 10g，生地黄 10g，木通 6g，萹蓄 10g，小蓟 10g，白花蛇舌草 30g，竹叶 10g，猪苓 15g，生甘草 5g。7 剂，日 1 剂，水煎服。

Prescription: modified *Xiaoji Yinzi* Decoction.

Cheqiancao 15g, beishashen 20g, sigualuo 10g, shengdihuang 10g, mutong 6g, bianxu 10g, xiaoji 10g, baihuasheshecao 30g, zhuye 10g, zhuling 15g, shenggancao 5g.

Seven doses and one dose a day, decoction.

证候分析：久病及肾，肾阴不足，形体不充，见消瘦；虚热内扰，则心烦少寐；津伤则口干；湿热下注，阻滞气机，见小便赤涩痛不畅，甚至白色浑浊物从尿中排出，大便时溏不爽；舌质红，苔薄黄，脉沉细，乃湿热内蕴伴阴虚不足之征象。

Syndrome analysis: prolonged illness affects the kidney and consumes kidney yin, which causes the body unfilled with blood and brings about emaciation. Internal disturbance of deficiency heat causes vexation and less sleep. Body fluid impairment results to dry mouth. Dampness-heat pouring downward blocks qi movement, causing red unsmooth painful urination with white turbidity, and unsmooth defecation with loose stool. Red tongue with thin yellow fur and deep thin pulse are manifestations of internal accumulation of dampness-heat accompanied with yin deficiency.

2009 年 9 月 25 日二诊：小便赤涩、白色浊物已无，不畅症状较前减轻，口稍干，精神好转，舌红，苔薄白（图 3.2.5.6b），脉沉细。前方加女贞子、墨旱莲草 15g，五味子 10g，7 剂。诸症明显好转。

Second visit on September 25, 2009: red urination with white turbidity was removed and unsmooth urination alleviated. The mouth was slightly dry and the spirit was getting better. The patient had red tongue with thin white fur (Fig.3.2.5.6b) and deep thin pulse. Seven doses of the previous prescription were used for treatment with the addition of nüzhenzi 15g, mohanlian 15g, and wuweizi 10g. Then all symptoms were markedly improved.

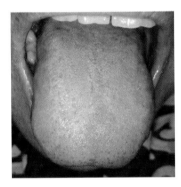 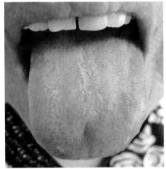

图 3.2.5.6a 图 3.2.5.6b
Fig.3.2.5.6a Fig.3.2.5.6b

（七）淋证 – 湿热内阻证

5.7 Stranguria: syndrome of internal obstruction of dampness-heat

患者申某，女，26 岁，已婚，反复小便涩痛 1 年，右下腹痛 3 个月，于 2015 年 4 月 21 日初诊。

Patient Shen, female, 26 years old, married, had been suffering from repeated unsmooth and painful urination for one year, with pain in the right lower abdomen for 3 months. She came to see the doctor on April 21, 2015.

患者于 1 年前游泳后出现尿频、尿急、尿痛等症状，当地医院诊为尿路感染，给予抗生素治疗，症状有所减轻。近 3 个月来，患者出现右下腹疼痛，遂来就诊。刻诊：小便时有尿道刺痛伴灼热感，无尿频、尿急，右下腹隐痛，纳可，睡眠佳，大便调。舌质红，少苔（图 3.2.5.7a），脉细弦。白带量稍多，外阴瘙痒（－）。月经史5～6/26～30 天，末次月经 2015 年 3 月 16 日，量正常，色红，血块（＋），经前乳房胀痛（＋），痛经（－），腰酸（－）。尿常规示：白细胞（＋＋＋）。腹部 B 超检查（－）。

The patient had frequent, urgent and painful urination after swimming one year ago. She was diagnosed as urinary tract infection (UTI) and treated by antibiotics, with the symptoms improved. In recent 3 months, she had pain in the right lower abdomen, so she came to see the doctor. Present symptoms: stabbing pain in urinary tract with burning sensation, no frequent and urgent urination, dull pain in the right lower abdomen, normal appetite, good sleep, normal stool, red tongue with scanty fur (Fig.3.2.5.7a), and thread wiry pulse, slightly profuse leucorrhea, pruritus vulvae (-). Menstrual history: 5-6/26-30 days, LMP: March 16, 2015, normal amount, red color, blood clot (+), pre-menstrual breast pain (+), dysmenorrhea (-), waist soreness (-). Routine urine test: white blood cells (+++). Abdominal B-ultrasound examination (-).

西医诊断：尿道炎。

Western medicine diagnosis: urethritis.

中医诊断：淋证。

TCM diagnosis: stranguria.

辨证：湿热内阻，气滞血瘀兼肾虚证。

Syndrome differentiation: internal obstruction of dampness-heat, qi stagnation and blood stasis accompanied with kidney deficiency.

治疗：清热利湿，行气化瘀止痛，佐以补肾固本。

Treatment: clearing heat and draining dampness, promoting qi, resolving stasis and relieving pain, as well as tonifying kidney and consolidating the root.

处方：八正散加减：车前草 15g，滑石 15g，萹蓄 10g，瞿麦 10g，川楝子 10g，醋延胡索 15g，丹参 15g，赤芍 15g，白花蛇舌草 30g，五灵脂 10g、蒲公英 15g，毛冬青 20g，桑寄生 30g，续断 15g。7 剂，日 1 剂，水煎服。

Prescription: modified *Bazheng* Powder.

Cheqiancao 15g, huashi 15g, bianxu 10g, qumai 10g, chuanlianzi 10g, yanhusuo 15g, danshen 15g, chishao 15g, baihuasheshecao 30g, wulingzhi 10g, pugongying 15g, maodongqing 20g, sangjisheng 30g, xuduan 15g.

Seven doses and one dose a day, decoction.

证候分析：湿热蕴结下焦，膀胱气化失司，故见小腹隐痛、小便灼热、短数；湿热内阻，血行不畅而成瘀，则见尿道刺痛；舌质红，少苔，脉细弦，为湿热内阻之征。

Syndrome analysis: dampness-heat accumulating in lower-energizer causes bladder's disorder of qi transformation, so dull pain in lower abdomen and scanty frequent urination with burning sensation appear. Internal obstruction of dampness-heat induces stagnation of blood, so stabbing pain in urinary tract appear. Red tongue with scanty fur and thready wiry pulse are the signs of internal obstruction of dampness-heat.

2015 年 4 月 28 日二诊：尿道灼热刺痛症状减轻，右下腹仍有隐痛，无腰酸，舌淡红，苔薄白（图 3.2.5.7b），脉弦细。原方加薏苡仁 20g、白茅根 20g、大腹皮 10g，继服 7 剂。

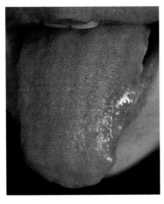 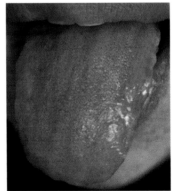

图 3.2.5.7a　　　　　　　　　图 3.2.5.7b
Fig.3.2.5.7a　　　　　　　　Fig.3.2.5.7b

Second visit on April 28, 2015: the symptoms of burning sensation and stabbing pain of urinary tract were alleviated, but dull pain in the right lower abdomen was not improved. There was no waist soreness, light red tongue with thin white fur (Fig.3.2.5.7b), and thready wiry pulse. Seven doses of the previous prescription were used for treatment, with the addition of yiyiren 20g, baimaogen 20g, and dafupi 10g.

2015 年 5 月 5 日三诊：患者精神佳，尿痛、腹痛等症状明显减轻，继服用贞芪扶正颗粒善后。

Third visit on May 5, 2015: the patient had normal spirit and the symptoms such as pain in urination and abdominal pain were alleviated. *Zhenqi Fuzheng Granule* was used for rehabilitation.

（八）石淋 – 湿热内蕴证
5.8 Stone stranguria: syndrome of dampness-heat accumulation

患者李某，男，48 岁，右侧腰部绞痛 1 日，于 2012 年 3 月 2 日就诊。

Patient Li, male, 48 years old, had been suffering from colic pain in the right lumbar for one day, so he came to see the doctor on March 2, 2012.

患者 1 天前突发右侧腰部绞痛,汗出伴呕吐,于当地医院就诊,B 超示"右肾积水,右肾肾盂壶腹部结石",肌注 654-2，症状缓解回家，后又剧痛，伴尿血，遂来就诊。刻诊：面色苍白,呻吟不已,汗出如珠,卷缩状,腰痛拒按,小便涩痛,尿中可见白浊物,舌红，苔黄腻（图 3.2.5.8a），脉弦数。尿常规检查示：红细胞（+++）。

The patient had a sudden colic pain in the right of waist, accompanied with sweating and vomiting one day ago and came to see the doctor in the local hospital. B-mode ultrasonography: right hydronephrosis and calculi in the right renal pelvis. He was injected with 654-2 and went back home with symptoms relieved. Severe pain and hematuria occur, so he came for treatment. Present symptoms: pale complexion, groaning incessantly, pearl-like sweating, curled body position, unpalpable abdominal pain, unsmooth painful urination with whitish turbidity, red tongue with yellow greasy fur (Fig.3.2.5.8a), and wiry rapid pulse. Routine urine test: RBC (+++).

西医诊断：肾结石。

Western medicine diagnosis: renal calculus.

中医诊断：石淋。

TCM diagnosis: stone stranguria.

辨证：湿热蕴结证。

Syndrome differentiation: dampness-heat accumulation.

治疗：清热利湿，通淋排石。

Treatment: clearing heat and draining dampness, relieving stranguria and expelling stone.

处方：四金汤加减：金钱草 30g，海金沙 15g，鸡内金 15g，郁金 10g，白芍 15g，小蓟 15g，延胡索 15g，地榆炭 15g，石韦 10g，白花蛇舌草 30g，滑石 20g，冬葵子 12g，泽泻 10g，通草 3g，琥珀末 3g（冲服）。2 剂，日 1 剂，水煎服。

Prescription: modified *Sijin* Decoction.

Jinqiancao 30g, haijinsha 15g, jineijin 15g, yujin 10g, baishao 15g, xiaoji 15g, yanhusuo 15g, diyutan 15g, shiwei 10g, baihuasheshecao 30g, huashi 20g, dongkuizi 12g, zexie 10g, tongcao 3g, hupomo3g (take medicine with water).

Two doses and one dose a day, decoction.

证候分析：湿热蕴结，煎浊尿液，凝为砂石；湿热阻滞尿道，则小便涩痛；湿热灼伤血络，见尿血；湿热蕴结腰府，阻滞气机，出现腰部绞痛；气机通降受阻，上逆而见呕吐；湿热熏蒸，则汗出如珠；舌红，苔黄腻，脉弦数，为湿热内蕴之征象。

Syndrome analysis: internal accumulation of dampness-heat causes urine calculus. Dampness-heat blocks urethra, so unsmooth painful urination happens. Dampness-heat burns the blood collaterals, leading to hematuria. Dampness-heat accumulates in the waist and blocks qi movement, which causes the colic pain in the waist. Qi moves upward and causes vomiting. Fumigation of dampness-heat leads to pearl-like sweating. The red tongue with yellow greasy fur and wiry rapid pulse are manifestations of internal accumulation of dampness-heat.

2012 年 3 月 4 日二诊：服药后腰部绞痛症状逐渐缓解，能忍受，尿色转清，舌淡、苔薄腻（图 3.2.5.8b），脉弦。上方继服 3 剂，巩固疗效。

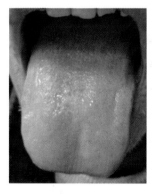 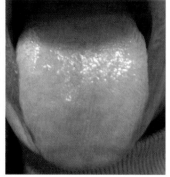

图 3.2.5.8a 图 3.2.5.8b
Fig.3.2.5.8a Fig.3.2.5.8b

Second visit on March 4, 2012: the colic pain in the waist was relieved and gradually turned to be tolerable pain after medication. The urine color turned clean. The tongue was pale with thin greasy fur (Fig.3.2.5.8b), and the pulse was wiry. Three doses of the original prescription were used to consolidate the efficacy.

（九）血淋－湿热下注证

5.9　Blood strangury: syndrome of dampness-heat flowing downward

患者蒋某，男，27 岁，小便热痛伴尿色深红 2 天，于 2016 年 7 月 15 日就诊。

Patient Jiang, male, 27 years old, had been suffering from burning and painful urination with dark red urine for 2 days, then he came to see the doctor on July 15, 2016.

患者 2 天前因过食辛辣出现小便不畅，热涩疼痛，量少而尿色深红而来就诊。刻诊：面色潮红，焦虑貌，小便灼热刺痛，尿量少而色深红，口苦口渴，口中黏腻，纳可，心烦，梦多，大便溏而不爽，舌质红，苔黄（图 3.2.5.9a），脉滑数。尿常规示：红细胞（+++），白细胞（+），尿蛋白（－）。血常规示：白细胞计数 11.7×10^9/L，血红蛋白 12g/L。肾功能：尿素氮（－），肌酐（－）。

The patient had difficult, burning and painful urination with dark red scanty urine 2 days ago because of overeating spicy foods, so he came to visit the doctor. Present symptoms: flushed complexion, anxious appearance, urination with scorching pain, scanty urine with dark red color, bitterness in the mouth with thirst, sticky mouth, normal appetite, vexation, dreaminess, unsmooth defecation with loose stool, red tongue with yellow fur (Fig.3.2.5.9a), and slippery rapid pulse. Routine urine test: RBC (+++), WBC (+), urine protein (-). Blood routine test: WBC 11.7×10^9/L, Hb 12g/L. Renal function: BUN (-), Scr (-).

西医诊断：急性尿道炎。

Western medicine diagnosis: acute urethritis.

中医诊断：血淋

TCM diagnosis: blood stranguria.

辨证：湿热下注，迫血妄行证。

Syndrome differentiation: dampness-heat flowing downward with frenetic movement of the blood.

治疗：清热凉血通淋。

Treatment: clearing heat, cooling blood and relieving stranguria.

处方：小蓟饮子加减：小蓟 15g，淡竹叶 10g，藕节 10g，生地黄 30g，滑石 15g，百合 15g，木通 6g，炒蒲黄 12g，血余炭 15g，当归 6g，栀子 10g，炙甘草 6g。7 剂，日 1 剂，水煎服。

Prescription: modified *Xiaoji Yinzi* Decoction.

Xiaoji 15g, danzhuye 10g, oujie 10g, shengdihuang 30g, huashi 15g, baihe 15g, mutong 6g, chaopuhuang 12g, xueyutan 15g, danggui 6g, zhizi 10g, zhigancao 6g.

Seven doses and one dose a day, decoction.

证候分析：湿热下注膀胱，热盛伤络，迫血妄行，以致小便涩痛有血；血块阻塞尿路，故疼痛满急加剧；湿热上移，心火亢盛，扰乱心神，则可见心烦；舌质红、苔黄，脉滑数，为湿热证之象。

Syndrome analysis: dampness-heat flows downward to the bladder, burns the collaterals and causes frenetic movement of the blood, so unsmooth painful urination with blood occurs. The blood clots block the urinary tract, which aggravates the pain and urination frequency. Dampness-heat moving upward and heart fire disturbing the mind lead to vexation. Red tongue with yellow fur and slippery rapid pulse are manifestations of dampness-heat syndrome.

2016 年 7 月 22 日二诊：患者神清气爽，精神佳，小腹不胀痛，小便无涩痛、尿色清，大便通畅，舌淡红，苔白（图 3.2.5.9b），脉缓。嘱清淡饮食，少食辛辣厚味。

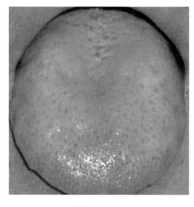
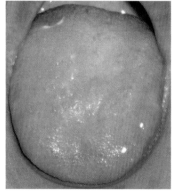

图 3.2.5.9a
Fig.3.2.5.9a

图 3.2.5.9b
Fig.3.2.5.9b

Second visit on July 15, 2016: the patient had good spirit, no distending pain in lower abdomen, no unsmooth painful urination, clear urine, normal stool, light red tongue with white fur (Fig.3.2.5.9b), and moderate pulse. The patient was advised to have light diet and less spicy and fat food.

（十）尿浊 – 脾肾气虚证

5.10　Turbid urine: syndrome of qi deficiency of spleen and kidney

患者柳某，男，53 岁，反复蛋白尿半年余，于 2015 年 11 月 3 日就诊。

Patient Liu, male, 53 years old, had been suffering from repeated proteinuria for half a year, so he came to see the doctor on November 3, 2015.

患者半年前因感冒在当地医院检查。尿常规示：尿蛋白（++），红细胞（ - ），白细胞（ - ）。肾功示：正常。B 超：双肾、输尿管、膀胱未见明显异常。患者间断服肾炎舒片治疗，近 1 个月来因腰酸乏力而就诊。刻诊：精神可，双肺及心脏听诊正常，肾区叩击痛（ - ），病理征（ - ），腰酸乏力，颜面无水肿，双下肢轻度浮肿，纳可，大便偏干，小便泡沫多，颜色正常，寐可，舌质淡，苔薄白（图 3.2.5.10a），脉弦细。尿常规：尿蛋白（+++），红细胞（ - ），白细胞（ - ）。

The patient was examined in the local hospital 6 months ago due to a cold. Routine urine test: urine protein (++), RBC (-), WBC (-). Renal function: normal. B-ultrasound: no obvious abnormalities in the kidneys, ureters and bladder. He was administered *Shenyanshu* Tablet intermittently for treatment. He came to see the doctor due to waist soreness and lassitude for a month. Present symptoms: normal spirit, normal auscultation in both lungs and heart, percussion pain in kidney area (-), pathological signs (-), soreness and weakness of waist , no facial edema, mild edema in the lower limbs, normal appetite, slightly dry stool, urine with profuse foam and normal color, normal sleep, pale tongue with thin white fur (Fig.3.2.5.10a), and wiry thready pulse. Routine urine test: urine protein (+++), RBC (-), WBC (-).

西医诊断：慢性肾炎。

Western medicine diagnosis: chronic nephritis.

中医诊断：尿浊。

TCM diagnosis: turbid urine.

辨证：脾肾气虚，精气不守证。

Syndrome differentiation: spleen-kidney qi deficiency and insecureness of essential qi.

治疗：健脾益肾，固精止遗。

Treatment: invigorating spleen and replenishing kidney, securing essence and stopping spermatorrhea.

处方：四君子汤加减：黄芪 15g，党参 10g，炒白术 10g，茯苓 15g，金樱子 20g，杜仲 15g，续断 15g，石韦 10g，马鞭草 15g，鬼箭羽 20g，玉米须 15g，炒薏苡仁 20g，白豆蔻 10g，蝉衣 6g，芡实 10g，垂盆草 15g。14 剂，日 1 剂，水煎服。

Prescription: modified *Sijunzi* Decoction.

Huangqi 15g, dangshen 10g, chaobaizhu 10g, fuling 15g, jinyingzi 20g, duzhong 15g, xuduan 15g, shiwei 10g, mabiancao 15g, guijianyu 20g, yumixu 15g, yiyiren 20g, baidoukou 10g, chanyi 6g, qianshi 10g, chuipencao 15g.

Fourteen doses and one dose a day, decoction.

证候分析：腰为肾之府，肾气不足，腰府失养，而见腰酸乏力；肾气不足，气化失职，水液不循常道，泛溢肌肤而见腰府以下肿；脾虚升清受损，肾虚封藏失职，而见小便尿浊、泡沫多；舌质淡，苔薄白，脉弦细，乃脾肾气虚，化源不足，不能充养之明证。

Syndrome analysis: the waist is the house of the kidney, and the insufficiency of kidney qi fails to nourish the waist, so waist soreness and lassitude appear. Insufficiency of kidney qi causes the dysfunction of qi transformation, which induces water-fluid flowing abnormally to overflow into the skin, so edema below the waist appears. Spleen deficiency failing to ascend the clear and kidney deficiency failing to store essence explains turbid urine with profuse foam. Light tongue with thin white fur and wiry thready pulse are the signs of qi deficiency of spleen and kidney with insufficient generation and transformation as well as nourishment.

2015 年 11 月 10 日二诊：患者自觉腰酸症状减轻。尿常规：尿蛋白（++），红细胞 0 ～ 1 个 /HP，白细胞（－）。舌质淡红，苔薄白（图 3.2.5.10b），脉细。上方去续断，加牛膝 20g，14 剂。

Second visit on November 10, 2015: the symptom of waist soreness was alleviated. Routine urine test: urine protein (++), RBC 0-1/HP, WBC (-). Light red tongue with thin white fur (Fig. 3.2.5.10b), and wiry pulse. Fourteen doses of the original prescription were modified for treatment, with the removal of xuduan and the addition of niuxi 20g.

2015 年 11 月 25 日三诊：患者自觉症状缓解，24 小时尿蛋白 0.573g。尿常规：尿蛋白（＋），红细胞（－），白细胞（－）。各项指标趋于正常，继续守方，以巩固疗效。

Third visit on November 25, 2015: the symptoms were relieved, urine protein in 24 hours was 0.573g. Routine urine test: urine protein (+), RBC (-), WBC (-). The indicators was tending to be normal. Therefore, the original prescription was used to consolidate the effect.

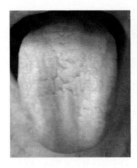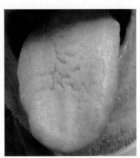

图 3.2.5.10a　　　　图 3.2.5.10b
Fig.3.2.5.10a　　　　Fig.3.2.5.10b

（十一）消渴 – 肾阴亏虚证

5.11　Consumptive thirst: syndrome of kidney yin deficiency

患者程某，男，48 岁，多饮多尿乏力 5 年加重 2 月，于 2015 年 4 月 5 日就诊。

Patient Cheng, male, 48 years old, had been suffering from polydipsia, polyuria and fatigue for 5 years and the symptoms aggravated for 2 months, so he came to see the doctor on April 5, 2015.

患者 5 年前因多饮多尿乏力于当地医院诊为 2 型糖尿病，口服二甲双胍片等降糖药物治疗，但效果欠佳。近 2 月来口渴多饮症状加重而来就诊。刻诊：精神倦怠，形体消瘦，腰背酸软，夜寐梦多，小便频，大便干，舌质暗红，苔黄干（图 3.2.5.11a），右脉沉细，左脉小弦数。查血糖 15.80mmol/L，尿糖（＋＋＋）。

The patient was diagnosed as diabetes (type 2) by the local hospital 5 years ago for the symptoms of polydipsia, polyuria and fatigue. He was treated with hypoglycemic drugs such as metformin tablets, without good effect. In the past 2 months, thirst and polydipsia have worsened, so he came to see the doctor. Present symptoms: fatigue, emaciation, aching and weak waist and back, dreaminess, frequent urination, dry stool, dark red tongue with yellow dry fur (Fig.3.2.5.11a), deep thready pulse in the right hand and wiry rapid pulse in the left. Blood glucose was 15.80 mmol/L and urine sugar (++).

西医诊断：糖尿病。

Western medicine diagnosis: diabetes.

中医诊断：消渴。

TCM diagnosis: consumptive thirst.

辨证：肾阴亏虚，津液不足证。

Syndrome differentiation: kidney yin deficiency and body fluid insufficiency.

治疗：滋补肝肾，益气养阴。

Treatment: nourishing kidney and liver, replenishing qi and nourishing yin.

处方：知柏地黄汤加减：黄芪 15g，怀山药 15g，地锦草 30g，山茱萸 15g，天花粉 15g，生地黄 15g，麦冬 12g，茯苓 15g，泽泻 15g，牡丹皮 10g。7 剂，日 1 剂，水煎服。

Prescription: modified *Zhibai Dihuang* Decoction.

Huangqi 15g, huaishanyao 15g, dijincao 30g, shanzhuyu 15g, tianhuafen 15g, shengdihuang 15g, maidong 12g, fuling 15g, zexie 15g, mudanpi 10g.

Seven doses and one dose a day, decoction.

证候分析：肾阴亏虚日久，阴不制阳，虚阳浮越，消灼津液而致口苦口渴；阴亏，形体不充则消瘦；肾阴亏虚，腰府失养，则腰背酸痛；阴虚内热，上扰心神，则失眠；肾失固涩，水精下注，则小便频数；阴虚血涩，则见舌红暗，少苔，脉细数。

Syndrome analysis: chronic deficiency of kidney yin and yin failing to restrain yang cause upward floating of deficiency yang, which scorches body fluid and induces thirst and bitterness in the mouth. Insufficiency of yin fails to nourish the body, so emaciation appears. Insufficiency of kidney yin fails to nourish the waist, so aching pain of the waist and back appear. Yin deficiency and endogenous heat disturbs the mind upward, thus insomnia appears. Kidney failing to secure essence causes water and essence to pour downward, so frequent urination appears. Dark red tongue with scanty fur and thready rapid pulse are the signs of yin deficiency and blood roughness.

2015 年 4 月 12 日二诊：口苦口渴症状减轻，小便减少，但仍有腰背酸软，夜寐梦多，舌暗红，苔黄腻（图 3.2.5.11b），脉细弦。上方加茯神 20g、牛膝 20g，继服 14 剂。

Second visit on April 12, 2015: thirst and bitterness in the mouth were alleviated and the frequency of urination was reduced. But there were still symptoms of aching and weak waist and back, dreaminess, dark red tongue with yellow greasy fur (Fig.3.2.5.11b), and thready wiry pulse. 14 doses of the original prescription were used for further treatment, with the addition of fushen 20g and niuxi 20g.

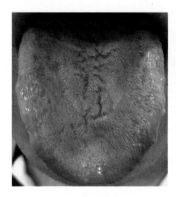 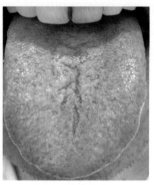

图 3.2.5.11a   图 3.2.5.11b
Fig.3.2.5.11a   Fig.3.2.5.11b

2015 年 4 月 28 日三诊：复查血糖 8.6mmol/L，尿糖（±），服用知柏地黄丸善后，病情平稳。

Third visit on April 28, 2015: blood glucose: 8.6mmol/L; urine sugar (±). *Zhibai Dihuang* Pill was used for rehabilitation.

（十二）消渴 – 肾阴阳两虚证

5.12 Consumptive thirst: syndrome of deficiency of both yin and yang of kidney

患者张某，男，71 岁，发现血糖高、肾功能异常 5 年，咳嗽咯痰、胸闷 1 个月，于 2015 年 11 月 21 日就诊。

Patient Zhang, male, 71 years old, had been suffering from hyperglycemia and abnormal renal function for 5 years. In recent one month, he had cough, expectoration and chest tightness, so he came to see the doctor on November 21, 2015.

患者于 5 年前诊断为 2 型糖尿病，半年前出现四肢麻木、蚁行感，偶有针扎样刺痛感，伴头晕、头痛、胸闷不适。1 个月前患者无明显诱因出现咳嗽咯痰、胸闷，遂来就诊。刻诊：精神差，全身瘙痒，咳嗽、咯痰，胸闷、心慌，纳眠差，大便隔日一行，色黑，小便量可，夜尿多，约 1000mL，舌淡红，苔稍黄干（图 3.2.5.12a），脉沉细稍无力。肾功能：尿素氮 28.2mmol/L，肌酐 642.7μmol/L，尿酸 422μmol/L。

The patient was diagnosed as diabetes (type 2) 5 years ago. Half a year ago, he felt numbness, formication, and occasional stinging pain in the limbs, accompanied by dizziness, headache, and chest tightness. One month ago, the patient had cough, expectoration and chest tightness without obvious inducement, so he came to see the doctor. Present symptoms: dispiritedness, general itching, cough, expectoration, chest tightness, flusteredness, poor appetite and sleep, defecation once every other day with black stool, normal urine, frequent night urination with about 1000mL/day, light red tongue with slightly yellow dry fur (Fig.3.2.5.12a), deep, thready and slightly weak pulse. Renal function: BUN 28.2 mmol/L, Scr 642.7 μmol/L, UA 422 μmol/L.

西医诊断：慢性肾衰竭；2 型糖尿病肾病。

Western medicine diagnosis: chronic renal failure; diabetic nephropathy (type 2).

中医诊断：消渴 – 下消。

TCM diagnosis: consumptive thirst (lower consumption).

辨证：阴阳两虚，阴津不固证。

Syndrome differentiation: deficiency of both yin and yang with insecure fluid.

治疗：滋阴补阳，益气养阴。

Treatment: nourishing yin, tonifying yang, and replenishing qi.

处方：自拟方：黄芪 30g，山药 20g，炙黄精 20g，石韦 15g，泽泻 15g，龟甲 20g，当归 20g，土茯苓 15g，锁阳 15g，款冬花 15g，桔梗 10g，杏仁 10g，砂仁 6g，山楂 15g，肉苁蓉 15g。7 剂，日 1 剂，水煎服。

Prescription: self-formulated prescription.

Huangqi 30g, shanyao 20g, zhihuangjing 20g, shiwei 15g, zexie 15g, guijia 20g, danggui 20g, tufuling 15g, suoyang 15g, kuandonghua 15g, jiegeng 10g, xingren 10g, sharen 6g, shanzha 15g, roucongrong 15g.

Seven doses and one dose a day, decoction.

证候分析：患者久病，阴损及阳，阴阳俱虚，阳虚机体失于气化、温养，可见四肢麻木、蚁行感，伴头晕、头痛、胸闷不适等症；肾阴阳两虚，开阖失职，固摄无权，可见尿频；舌淡红，苔稍黄干，提示正气不足，邪郁化热之象；脉沉细而无力，则为阴阳俱虚，脉道失充，无力推动之象。

Syndrome analysis: prolonged illness and detriment of yin affecting yang cause both deficiency of yin and yang. Yang deficiency causes dysfunction of qi transformation, warming and nourishing, therefore the symptoms such as numbness of the limbs, formication, dizziness, headache, chest tightness appear. Both deficiency of yin and yang of kidney causes dysfunction in opening, closing and consolidating, so frequent urination appears. Light red tongue with slightly yellow dry fur indicates that healthy qi is insufficient and pathogenic depression transforms into heat. Deep, thready and weak pulse reflects both deficiency of yin and yang, which causes unfilled vessels and weak propelling of qi.

2015 年 11 月 28 日二诊：咳嗽、咳痰、胸闷症状减轻，寐差，夜尿多，大便可，舌淡红，苔白干（图 3.2.5.12b），脉沉。原方加益智仁 20g、五味子 10g、夜交藤 30g。

Second visit on November 28, 2015: the syndromes of cough, expectoration and chest tightness had been alleviated. There were symptoms of poor sleep, frequent night urination, normal stool, light red tongue with white dry fur (Fig.3.2.5.12b), and deep pulse. The original prescription was used for treatment, with the addition of yizhiren 20g, wuweizi 10g, and yejiaoteng 30g.

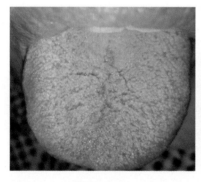 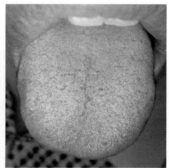

图 3.2.5.12a
Fig.3.2.5.12a

图 3.2.5.12b
Fig.3.2.5.12b

第四章　舌诊研究进展

Chapter 4　Research Progress of the Tongue Diagnosis

舌诊是中医望诊的重要内容之一，被历代医家所重视。人体五脏六腑、四肢百骸通过经络的络属关系与舌体构成一个有机的整体，脏腑的生理功能、病理变化可通过舌的动态变化反映出来，因此舌质、舌苔、舌态及舌下络脉的变化是中医辨证论治的重要医学依据。当今，现代科技的发展及在医学领域中的广泛运用促使中医舌诊开展了多角度研究。

Tongue diagnosis is one of the important contents of the inspection diagnoses of TCM, which has always been valued by doctors through all ages. The five zang-organs and six fu-organs, four limbs and skeleton and tongue body form an organic whole through the relationship of channel and collateral. The physiological function and pathological change of *zang-fu* organs can be reflected by the dynamic changes of the tongue. Therefore, the changes of tongue body, tongue fur, tongue motility, and sublingual collaterals are the important medical basis of TCM syndrome differentiation and treatment. Nowadays, the development of modern science and technology and the extensive application in the medical field promote multi-angle research of the tongue diagnosis of Traditional Chinese Medicine.

第一节 舌诊临床应用研究

Section 1 Research on the Clinical
Application of Tongue Diagnosis

一、舌诊在肝系疾病中的应用

1. Application of tongue diagnosis in liver diseases

《灵枢·经脉》云："肝者筋之合也，筋者聚于阴器，而脉络于舌本也。"表明舌与肝存在内在关联性，舌的变化是肝病辨治的重要依据之一。

The Spiritual Pivot-Meridians said that "The Liver is related to the tendons which converge around the external genitalia and the channel links with the tongue root." It showed that the tongue and Liver had intrinsic correlation, and the change of tongue was one of the important evidences for the differentiation and treatment of Liver diseases.

许颖等改变传统望诊的宏观性，采用光谱测色法对原发性肝癌患者进行舌色数据分析，结果发现在原发性肝癌的四种不同证型中，舌色的色度坐标分布不同，存在明显色差，为肝癌规范化、标准化辨证分型提供了客观依据。赵丰润采用舌象仪对乙型肝炎肝硬化代偿期患者中医药干预前后舌色进行比较，根据舌色的 R、G、B、V 值的客观变化确定临床药物干预的效果，从舌色参数的量化来佐证药物疗效的确切性。

Xu Ying, etc. changed the macro of traditional inspection and used spectral color measurement method for data analysis on the tongue color of patients with primary hepatocellular carcinoma. It was found that in four different kinds of syndromes of primary hepatocellular carcinoma, the color distribution of tongue color was different, and there was obvious chromatic aberration, which provided objective basis for the standardization of syndrome differentiation of liver cancer. Using tongue manifestation instrument to compare tongue color before and after Chinese medicine intervention in patients with hepatitis B cirrhosis, and according to the objective changes of R, G, B and V of tongue color, Zhao Fengrun determined the effect of clinical drug intervention, and confirmed the accuracy of drug efficacy from the quantification of tongue color parameters.

宫爱民等应用数字化四诊仪采集肝纤维化患者在不同证型中的舌象信息，发现在不同证型中的舌色指数、苔色指数、胖瘦指数、厚薄指数各不相同，这些不同指数是临床辨证客观化、定量化及诊断治疗的重要依据。肝纤维化可引起肝血流的改变，表现在门静脉的迂曲及血流速度的变化，同时也可波及于舌下络脉。贾梓等对慢性乙肝肝纤维化程度与舌下络脉积分进行分析，发现慢性乙肝肝纤维化患者舌下络脉迂曲、瘀斑，其程度与门静脉内径大小、肝脏硬度指数呈正相关，从而证明舌下脉络迂曲扩张程度可作为肝纤维化临床诊断的重要指标。

Gong Aimin, etc. collected tongue manifestation information of Liver fibrosis patients in different syndromes with digital four examinations instrument and found that the tongue color index, the tongue fur color index, the fat-thin index and the thick-thin index of different syndromes were all different, which were the important basis for the objective, quantitative and diagnostic treatment of clinical syndrome differentiation. Hepatic fibrosis can cause changes of hepatic blood flow, which is manifested in the changes of portal vein and blood flow velocity, and can also affect sublingual vein. Jia Zi, etc. analyzed the degree of chronic hepatitis B liver fibrosis and the integral of sublingual vein, and found that the extent of the sublingual vein tortuous and ecchymosis in patients with chronic hepatitis B liver fibrosis was positively correlated with the diameter of portal vein and the index of liver hardness, which proved that the extent of sublingual vein tortuous expansion could be used as an important index for clinical diagnosis of hepatic fibrosis.

疾病是动态变化的过程，在这个过程中，舌象是辨别疾病轻重、预后的重要指标。宋铭悦通过对舌象的动态变化与慢性重型肝炎肝胆湿热证患者的预后的相关性研究，发现舌象的动态变化、症状体征、生化指标的变化对慢性重型黄疸型肝炎患者的预后有较大程度的预测作用，对临床慢性重型肝炎的诊断、治疗及预后判断有重要价值。

Disease is the process of dynamic change, in which the tongue manifestation is an important indicator of the severity and prognosis of the disease. Song Mingyue, through the correlation study between dynamic changes of tongue manifestation and the prognosis of patients with syndrome of dampness-heat in chronic severe hepatitis, found that the dynamic changes of tongue manifestation and the changes of symptoms and sign as well as biochemical index had a greater degree of predictive effect on the prognosis of the patient with chronic severe jaundice hepatitis, which has great value to the diagnosis, treatment and prognosis of chronic severe hepatitis.

二、舌诊在心系疾病的应用
2. Application of tongue diagnosis in heart diseases

《灵枢·经脉》曰："手少阴之别……循经入于心中，系舌本。"心之络脉与舌直接相连。《素问·阴阳应象大论》曰："心主脉……在窍为舌。"舌的血络最为丰富，与心主血脉功能相关。《临症验舌法》曰："舌者，心之苗也。"指出舌为心之苗窍，与心的生理功能、病理变化直接相关。

The Spiritual Pivot-Meridians recorded that "The divergence of heart meridian of hand-shaoyin... goes through the heart and links with the tongue." *Plain Question- Treatise on Yin and Yang* recorded that "Heart dominates vessels...opens into tongue." The abundant tongue vessels are related to its function of controlling blood and vessels. *Tongue Diagnosis for Clinical Practice* said that "The tongue is the signal orifices of the heart." It was pointed out that tongue is the signal orifices of the heart, which is directly related to the physiological function and pathological changes of the heart.

李晓东等对 151 例冠心病患者进行舌象观察，发现所有患者舌下络脉均有不同程度的扩张、扭曲或瘀斑，表明瘀血阻滞是冠心病的主要病机；另外，有 1/3 患者的舌苔为白腻或黄腻，提示痰浊阻滞是冠心病的又一重要病机；另有 1/3 患者在急性心肌梗死发病前出现了舌尖小块剥落现象，且血清酶学检查发现此类患者的肌酸磷酸激酶值较非剥斑者为高，提示心肌梗死范围较大，坏死心肌数目多，认为舌象变化在临床上可作为心肌梗死辨别的一个重要警示指标。

Li Xiaodong, etc. observed the tongue manifestation of 151 patients with coronary heart disease, and found that all the patients had different degrees of dilation, distortion or ecchymosis of the sublingual collaterals, which indicated that static blood was the main pathogenesis of coronary heart disease. In addition, 1/3 of the patients with white-greasy or yellow-greasy tongue fur suggested that turbid phlegm obstruction was another important pathogenesis of coronary heart disease.

Another 1/3 patients showed the spalling phenomenon of a small piece of tongue in acute myocardial infarction premorbid, and the serum enzyme examination found that this type of patient's creatine phosphokinase value was higher than that of the non-peel. It suggested that the range of myocardial infarction was larger, the number of necrotic myocardium was more, and the change of tongue manifestation in clinical can be used as an important warning indicator of myocardial infarction.

徐学功等对慢性心力衰竭患者的心功能分级与中医证型及舌象特点进行关联性分析，发现心功能Ⅱ级患者以气虚血瘀证为多，以淡红舌、红舌、薄白苔、舌下络脉淡紫色为主；心功能Ⅲ级者以气虚血瘀证居多，舌象以暗红舌、薄白苔、舌下络脉青紫为多见；而心功能Ⅳ级者以阳虚水泛夹痰瘀互阻证为多，舌象以暗红舌、白苔稍厚、舌下络脉青紫最为常见。这表明随着心功能分级的增加，患者的舌色由淡红逐渐向暗红转变，苔质由薄苔逐渐向稍厚苔转变，舌下络脉颜色由淡紫向青紫转变，提示舌象的变化可以作为心衰程度轻重的一个重要诊断指标。

Xu Xuegong, etc. analyzed the relationship between cardiac function grading and TCM syndromes and tongue manifestation characteristics in patients with chronic heart failure, and found that the patients of the heart function level Ⅱ with qi deficiency and blood stasis syndrome were more, and they mainly had light red tongue, red tongue, thin-white tongue fur, and sublingual veins pale purple, and that the patients of the heart function level Ⅲ with qi deficiency and blood stasis syndrome were more, and the tongue manifestation were mainly dark red tongue, thin-white tongue fur, and blue purple sublingual vein; however, the patients of the heart function Ⅳ level with edema due to yang deficiency and phlegm-blood stasis syndrome were more, and the tongue manifestation like dark red tongue, white slightly thick tongue fur, and blue purple sublingual vein were most common. The results showed that with the increase of cardiac function, the tongue color changed from light red to dark red, and the fur texture gradually changed from thin fur to slightly thick fur, and the color of the sublingual veins changed from purple to blue. It suggested that the change of tongue manifestation could be an important diagnostic index for the degree of the severity of heart failure.

赵志宏采用上海道生舌象仪分析不稳定型心绞痛重度心气虚证患者介入术前、术后 1 个月和 10 个月的舌象，根据舌象的变化，结合临床各项指标，认为舌象可以作为冠心病证候演变的客观依据。

Zhao Zhihong used Shanghai Dao-sheng Tongue manifestation instrument to analyze the tongue manifestation of patients with severe heart qi deficiency syndrome of unstable angina pectoris before interventional operation, and one months as well as 10 months after interventional operation. According to the changes of tongue manifestation and the clinical indexes, the tongue manifestation could be used as the objective basis for the syndrome evolution of coronary.

杨忠奇采用 16SrDNA 测序技术研究冠心病痰浊证患者舌苔菌群的构成，结果发现菌群 Bacteroidetes（拟杆菌门）、Bacteroidia（拟杆菌纲）、Bacteroidales（拟杆菌目）、Paraprevotellaceae（帕拉普氏菌科）、Prevotellaceae（普雷沃氏菌科）、Prevotella（普雷沃氏菌属）在冠心病（痰浊证）组中丰度明显高于健康对照组，且上述菌群在两组间丰度差异具有临床意义，提示上述菌群的过度繁殖可能与痰浊的形成相关。而菌群 Lactobacillaceae（乳酸杆菌科）、Lactobacillus（乳酸杆菌属）、Lactobacillus salivarius（唾液乳酸杆菌）在急性心肌梗死痰浊证组中较心绞痛痰浊证组含量较高，且上述菌群在两组间丰度差异可能具有临床意义，提示上述菌群可能与冠心病急性加重或冠脉堵塞相关，从而认为舌苔微生态状况是检测冠心病的一个客观指标。

Yang Zhongqi used 16SrDNA sequencing technique to study the composition of tongue fur flora in patients of coronary heart disease with phlegm-turbidity syndrome, and found that the abundance of Bacteroidetes, Bacteroidia, Bacteroidales, Paraprevotellaceae, Prevotellaceae and Prevotella in coronary heart disease (phlegm-turbidity syndrome) group was significantly higher than that in healthy control group, and that the difference of abundance between the two groups had clinically significant, which suggested that the overgrowth of these flora might be related to the formation of turbid phlegm. However, the flora of Lactobacillaceae, Lactobacillus and Lactobacillus-salivarius in the patients of acute myocardial infarction with phlegm-turbidity syndrome were higher than that in the patients of angina with phlegm-turbidity syndrome, and the difference of abundance between the two groups might have clinical significance. It suggested that the above flora may be related to the acute exacerbation of coronary heart disease or occlusion of coronary arteries, so the micro-ecological status of tongue fur is an objective index to detect coronary heart disease.

史益平也研究了冠心病患者的舌质变化，发现舌象的各种微妙变化能及时反映心脏各种生理功能和病理表现，对心脏疾病的诊断、治疗、预后等有重要的指导作用。

Shi Yiping has studied the changes of tongue texture in patients with coronary heart disease and found that the various subtle changes of tongue manifestation can reflect the physiological function and pathological manifestation of the heart in time, and have important guiding effect on the diagnosis, treatment and prognosis of heart disease.

三、舌诊在脾胃系疾病的应用
3. Application of tongue diagnosis in spleen-stomach diseases

足太阴之别连舌本，散舌下。舌为脾之外候，舌苔为胃气上蒸所致，故脾胃疾病最先在舌质与舌苔上表现。针对慢性胃炎方面，舌象与胃镜象有着高度的一致性。

The collateral stemming from the spleen channel of foot-taiyin reaches the root of the tongue and spreads over its lower surface. The tongue is the external manifestation of the spleen and the tongue fur is caused by the steaming up of stomach qi, so the spleen and stomach diseases are first manifested on the tongue texture and tongue fur. For chronic gastritis, the tongue manifestation and the gastroscope has highly consistence.

吴耀南、方华珍对慢性浅表性胃炎病例舌象特征进行证型分类，并观察其舌象特点和与 Hp 之间的联系。吴氏研究表明 Hp 的感染对患者舌象也有所影响，感染者舌色多为红色，舌下脉络多迂曲；未感染者舌色多为淡红色，舌下脉络迂曲较前者较少。方氏研究发现脾胃虚弱型以淡白舌多见，脾胃湿热型以红舌为主，胃阴不足型出现红舌或红绛舌，肝胃不和型可见淡红舌，胃络瘀血型见紫（暗）舌。而在疾病的早期或恢复期以薄白苔为主，若舌苔黄腻或变为灰黑苔，病情多属加重。其中灰黑苔、黄厚腻、白厚腻、薄黄、薄白苔患者 Hp 阳性率逐渐降低。针对广泛的胃部疾病，舌象依然有参考价值。

Wu Yaonan and Fang Huazhen classified the tongue manifestations of chronic superficial gastritis and observed the characteristics of tongue manifestations and the relationship with Hp. Wu's study showed that Hp infection also had some effects on the patient's tongue manifestations. The tongue color of infected people was mostly red and the sublingual veins were more tortuous. Whereas the tongue color of uninfected people was mostly pale red and the sublingual veins were less tortuous than those of the former. Fang's study found that the syndrome of spleen-stomach weakness was usually seen with more pale tongue; the syndrome of dampness-heat of spleen and stomach, with red tongue mainly; the syndrome of stomach yin deficiency, with red or crimson tongue; disharmony of liver and kidney, with pale red tongue; the syndrome of stasis in stomach collateral, with purple or dark tongue. The early or recovery period of the disease is mainly thin white fur, and if the fur is yellow greasy or turned into gray black, the disease is more severe. The positive rate of Hp in patients with gray black fur, yellow thick greasy fur, white thick greasy fur, thin yellow fur and thin white fur gradually decreased. The tongue manifestation still has reference value for extensive stomach diseases.

卢亚娟对 113 例患有胃部疾病的患者舌象观察，发现随着胃部疾病的轻重程度不同，舌象有所不同。随着胃部疾病的加重，舌苔逐渐由白转为黄，由薄转厚，而在疾病逐渐恢复时则相反；舌质亦随病情的加重，逐渐由淡红色转为红色。

Lu Yajuan observed the tongue manifestation of 113 patients with gastric disease, and found that the tongue manifestation were different with the severity of stomach disease, with the stomach disease aggravated, the fur gradually changed from white to yellow, from thin to thick, but when the disease gradually recovered, the situation was opposite. The tongue texture also gradually changed from pale red to red with the aggravation of the disease.

四、舌诊在肺系疾病的应用

4. Application of tongue diagnosis in lung diseases

肺通调水道，辅助运行一身津液散布，而舌之荣枯可反映一身津液盈亏，故临床多可通过观其舌象来推断肺部疾病的证型。

Lung governs regulation of water passage and assists the distribution of the body fluid, and the tongue's flourishing or withering can be a reflection of body fluid's sufficiency and insufficiency. So in clinical, observing the tongue manifestation may infer the syndrome of lung diseases.

安云霞等和张淑琴等观察痰热闭肺证肺炎患儿舌象及肺部啰音，结果表明，随着病情的逐步痊愈，舌苔由黄转薄白，舌质由红转为淡红。

An Yunxia, etc. and Zhang Shuqin, etc. observed the tongue manifestation and pulmonary rales of the syndrome of phlegm-heat obstructing lung in children with pneumonia, and the results showed that as the disease gradually recovered, the fur changed from yellow to thin white and the tongue body from red to pale red.

戴芳等研究了 7680 例当代名医医案和 1018 例临床案例，发现舌象中红舌、黄苔与白苔出现次数最多。在双层频权剪叉运算中，红舌、黄苔与白苔三者对肺部的诊断权值最大。腻苔出现频率虽不及前三者，但在该运算中诊断权值也较高，临床意义较大。

Dai Fang, etc. studied 7680 cases of contemporary famous doctors' medical cases and 1018 cases of clinical cases, and found that the red tongue with yellow fur and white fur appeared most frequently in tongue manifestation. In the double frequency weight shearing operation, the red tongue, the yellow fur and the white fur were the biggest diagnostic weights. Although the frequency of greasy fur was less than the first three, the value of diagnosis in this operation was also higher and the clinical significance was larger.

苏婉等对 207 例肺癌患者舌象在不同临床因素中的分布规律进行了研究，发现鳞癌患者主要以白腻、黄腻苔为主，腺癌患者以薄白苔占多数，早期肺癌患者以薄白苔多见，而晚期则多以白厚腻苔和黄腻苔为主，认为舌诊对肺癌中医辨证有着十分重要的意义，对观察患者病势进展亦具有一定的指导作用。

Su Wan, etc. had studied on correlation between different clinical factors and tongue image in 207 cases of lung cancer patients and found that the squamous lung cancer patients mainly had white greasy and yellow greasy fur while adnocarcinoma patients, thin white coating. Lung cancer patients' tongue in early stage was mainly thin white coating, while in late stage was mainly white thick greasy coating and yellow greasy coating. They believes that tongue diagnosis has great significance for syndrome differentiation and disease condition observation.

中医认为疾病因地而异，高振等通过舌脉来对比新疆与内地慢性阻塞性肺疾病（COPD）的区别，研究结果表明，新疆 COPD 较内地多阳虚而寒和燥邪伤津的表现。

其白苔与薄苔较内地为多，内地多见黄苔和腻苔；舌质瘀斑内地多于新疆，但紫舌新疆则多于内地。

Traditional Chinese Medicine believes that diseases vary from place to place. Gao Zhen, etc. compared the tongue manifestation and vessel difference of chronic obstructive pulmonary disease (COPD) between Xinjiang and inland area. The results showed that COPD in Xinjiang was more yang deficiency with cold and dryness damaging body fluid than in the inland. In Xinjiang, white fur and thin fur were more, while yellow fur and greasy fur were more in the inland; ecchymosis in the inland was more than in Xinjiang, while purple tongue in Xinjiang was more than in the inland.

五、舌诊在肾系疾病的应用

5. Application of tongue diagnosis in kidney diseases

张昱等观察了慢性肾功能衰竭维持性血透患者的舌象与血清超敏 C- 反应蛋白（hs-CRP）的关系，发现瘀血舌组的血清 hs-CRP 明显高于非瘀血舌组，认为瘀血舌可作为一种判断慢性肾功能衰竭疾病的潜在危险指标。

Zhang Yu, etc. observed the relationship between tongue manifestation and serum hs-CRP in patients with chronic renal failure, and found that the serum hs-CRP of blood stasis tongue group was higher than that of non-blood stasis tongue group, and thought that the blood stasis tongue could be regarded as a potential risk index for the diagnosis of chronic renal failure.

朱穆朗玛等在对比 157 例慢性肾病患者舌象参数的研究中发现，随着慢性肾病病情的加重，R、G、B、L 值明显逐渐降低，舌苔也逐渐变为腐腻，舌苔剥落程度加重，提示随着慢性肾病的加重，患者体内痰浊病理产物逐渐增加，气血严重亏虚，认为舌象的变化能为慢性肾功能衰竭的临床诊断提供客观依据。

In the study of tongue manifestation parameters in 157 patients with chronic nephropathy, Zhumulangma, etc. found that with the aggravation of chronic kidney disease, R, G, B, L value obviously and gradually reduced, the tongue fur also and gradually became curdy-greasy, and tongue fur peeling degree aggravated, which suggested that, with the aggravation of chronic kidney disease, the patient's pathological product of phlegm turbidity gradually increased and his/her qi and blood were seriously deficient. It was believed that the change of tongue manifestation can provide an objective basis for clinical diagnosis of chronic renal failure.

汤倩珏研究发现肝郁肾虚型慢性盆腔炎患者舌象在裂纹指数、厚薄指数、胖瘦指数、瘀斑指数上与正常人相比，差异有统计学意义；在胖瘦指数上，肝郁肾虚型与非肝郁肾虚型差异有统计学意义，治疗后胖瘦指数明显上升，瘀斑指数明显下降。故其认为慢性盆腔炎的辨证分型与舌象指数存在一定的关联性。而中医药治疗后，肝郁肾虚型患者的舌象指数（胖瘦指数、瘀斑指数）发生了较为明显的变化，舌象对临床疗效的观察也有一定的指导意义。

Tang qianjue found that in patients with chronic pelvic inflammatory disease with liver depression and kidney deficiency syndrome, the fissured tongue index, the thick-thin index, the enlarged-thin index and the ecchymosis index were statistically significant compared with those of normal people. On the enlarged-thin index, there was a statistically significant difference between the liver depression and kidney deficiency syndrome and other syndromes, with the enlarged-thin index increased obviously and the blood-stasis index decreased obviously after treatment. It was concluded that the syndrome differentiation of chronic pelvic inflammatory disease and tongue manifestation index had certain correlation. The tongue manifestation index (the enlarged-thin index, the ecchymosis index) of the patients with liver depression and kidney deficiency syndrome was changed obviously after the treatment with Traditional Chinese Medicine, therefore, the tongue manifestation had a certain guiding significance to the observation of clinical curative effect.

安鹏等通过对比 300 例原发性肾小球病患者舌象观察，发现胖大舌多出现在原发性肾小球病的脾肾气虚证、脾肾阳虚证、肺肾气虚证中，而瘦舌则多出现在肝肾阴虚证、气阴两虚证中；舌苔湿在脾肾气虚证、脾肾阳虚证、肺肾气虚证中多见，而苔干则在湿热证及瘀血证中多见，这与传统的中医辨证论治相一致。

An Peng, etc. compared the tongue manifestation of 300 cases of primary glomerular disease, and found that enlarged tongue was mainly appeared in the current primary glomerular disease of spleen-kidney qi deficiency syndrome, spleen-kidney yang deficiency syndrome, lung-kidney qi deficiency syndrome, and the thin tongue was mainly appeared in liver-kidney yin deficiency syndrome, qi-yin deficiency syndrome; wet tongue fur was more common in spleen-kidney qi deficiency syndrome, spleen-kidney yang deficiency syndrome, lung-kidney deficiency syndrome, but the dry tongue fur was mainly appeared in dampness-heat syndrome and blood stasis syndrome, which is consistent with TCM syndrome differentiation and treatment.

第二节 舌诊的实验研究

Section 2 Experimental Research of Tongue Diagnosis

随着中医诊断学的进一步发展，我们对舌诊的研究也不断地深入，各种实验研究和客观化研究层出不穷。近年来随着计算机技术飞速发展，舌诊研究利用该领域的技术做出了不少成果。同时，舌诊的实验方法也拓展出很多新的路径。

With the further development of diagnostics of Traditional Chinese Medicine, the research of tongue diagnosis is deepening and various experimental studies and objective studies are emerging. With the rapid development of computer technology in recent years, tongue diagnosis research based on the field of technology has made a lot of achievements. At the same time, the experimental method of tongue diagnosis has developed many new paths.

一、科学仪器的检测研究

1. Detection research of scientific instruments

其包括使用热像仪测定舌面温度场，通过计算生物传热得知内部温度等参数来量化舌诊信息的研究；B型超声测量舌的外形和舌体内血管等数据来判断血瘀证及鉴别诊断方面的研究；应用光学显微镜和电子显微镜观察齿痕舌周围组织和细胞形态的研究；通过激光共聚焦显微镜观察不同浓度的表皮生长因子（EGF）对舌鳞癌细胞胞内钙离子动态变化的影响；其他舌诊研究内容，例如舌体测算、舌色检查和津液测定仪器等。

It contains using the thermal imager to measure the surface temperature field of the tongue, quantifying the information of tongue diagnosis by calculating biological heat transfer to get some parameters such as the internal temperature; the study of B-ultrasonic in measuring the tongue form and blood vessel in the tongue to judge blood stasis syndrome and make differential diagnosis; the study on the morphology of the tissues and cells around the teeth-marked tongue mark by using optical microscope and electron microscope; using laser confocal microscopy to observe the effect of different concentrations of EGF on the dynamic changes of the intracellular calcium ions of SqCa cell; and other research contents of tongue diagnosis, such as tongue body measurement, tongue color check and body fluid measuring instrument and so on.

二、分子生物学技术的舌诊研究

2. Tongue diagnosis research of molecular biology technique

其包括通过分析血液红细胞压积、全血黏度等 7 项指标与血液流变学关系研究舌象变化；分析幽门螺杆菌阳性胃炎患者舌质、舌苔研究；帮助诊断临床某些疾病的研究，例如 pH 试纸测舌质、舌苔的 pH 值；舌诊的多样化研究，例如舌苔脱落细胞涂片、酸碱度检测、形态计量学检测等；运用 TUNEL 技术检测舌苔上皮细胞凋亡情况，分析舌苔变化原因的研究；应用表皮生长因子受体放射受体分析方法（RPA）分析舌苔、EGF-R 与肿瘤关系的研究；借助放射免疫技术，例如微量、小分子多肽等，研究不同人群舌苔形成与变化的关联。

It contains the study on the change of tongue manifestation by analyzing the relationship between 7 indexes of the blood (like blood hematocrit, whole blood viscosity) and hemorheology; the study on tongue texture and tongue fur in patients with helicobacter pylori positive gastritis; the study of the assistant diagnosis of certain clinical diseases, for example, the pH value of tongue texture and tongue fur by using pH test paper; the study on tongue diagnosis diversity, for example, tongue fur cast-off cells smear, pH value detection, morphometric detection, etc; the study on the detection of the apoptosis of tongue fur epithelial cells and the analysis of the causes of tongue fur change by TUNEL technique; the study on the relationship between tongue fur, EGF-R and tumor by using epidermal growth factor receptor radioreceptor assay analysis method (RPA); the study on the relationship between the formation and change of tongue fur in different populations by means of radiation immunological technique, such as trace amount and small molecular polypeptide etc.

中医认为舌苔的变化可反映胃气盛衰及邪气消长等情况，对中医辨证有重要意义。有研究表明表皮生长因子（EGF）可以通过 EGF-R 机制影响舌苔形成；有应用原位杂交、免疫组化和图像分析技术，检测舌苔舌上皮细胞凋亡及凋亡相关基因和蛋白产物的研究。这些研究方法在一定程度上能发现舌色、舌苔的病理机制，但研究对象单一，临床应用范围有限。

TCM believes that the changes of tongue fur can reflect the exuberance and decline of stomach qi, exuberance and debilitation of pathogenic qi, and has important significance for the syndrome differentiation of Traditional Chinese Medicine. Some studies have shown epidermal growth factor's influence on the formation of tongue fur through the mechanism of EGF-R; and the application of hybridization in situ, immune histochemical and image analysis techniques to detect the apoptosis and apoptosis-related genes and protein products of tongue epithelial cells. These methods can find the pathological mechanism of tongue color and tongue fur to some extent. But the research object is single and the scope of clinical application is limited.

三、光谱分析法

3. Spectral analysis method

利用多波长光谱数据对物质进行分析，可以更全面、客观地反映组织细胞的生理病理变化，以探寻不同个体之间的细微差别。根据物体反射率原理，物体对某波长光的反射率应是物体自身的物理特性，而不随光源光谱成分而变化。将光谱技术应用于舌诊中，既消除了主客观因素影响，又能更全面反映舌体信息，无疑为舌诊现代化开辟了新思路。

Using multi-wavelength spectral data to analyze the material can reflect the physiological and pathological changes of the tissue cells more comprehensively and objectively, and thus explore the subtle differences between different individuals. According to the principle of object reflectivity, the reflectivity of an object to a wavelength light should be the physical property of the object itself, and not changed with the change of the spectral composition of the light source. The application of spectral technique to tongue diagnosis not only eliminates the influence of subjective and objective factors, but also reflects the information of tongue body more comprehensively, which undoubtedly opens up a new idea for the modernization of tongue diagnosis.

单色仪采集舌苔颜色的反射光波长的实验说明舌质情况可被光谱分析所量化；利用红外技术测得患者舌体各个部分辐射强度不一的实验，部分证明舌体不同部分分候脏腑功能的客观性；基于光谱的舌色客观化方法，将光谱法用在舌色采集中，通过数据处理，排除背景噪声及操作过程中的各个不确定因素，从而降低对光源参数和采集方法的依赖性，更加准确、客观地反映舌象情况；通过采集表寒里热患者、健康人和风寒患者的舌反射光的光谱信息，发现光谱法可将健康人和表寒里热患者区分开，准确率达 85.6%，这为中医证型诊断提供了一种全新方法。对健康人和脂肪肝患者的舌尖光谱进行归一化反射率处理，并对未知健康人和脂肪肝患者的样本进行分类预测，其正确率达 89.7%；用同样方法对未知健康人和高黏血症患者的样本进行分类，正确率达 100%。其表明舌光谱分析能为疾病的辅助诊断提供依据。

An experiment collecting the wavelength of reflected light of tongue fur color by monochromator means that the information of tongue texture can be quantified by spectrum analysis. Using infrared technique to measure the different radiation intensity of each part of the tongue body proved that the objectivity of the different part of the tongue to manage the function of the *zang-fu* organs. The objectified method of tongue color based on spectroscopic methodology is used in tongue color collection. Through data processing and the elimination of background noise and various uncertain factors in operation process, the dependence on light source parameters and collection methods is reduced, and the tongue manifestation is reflected more accurately and objectively. By collecting the information of the tongue reflectance spectra of the patients with exterior cold and interior heat, the healthy and the wind-cold patients, we found that the spectroscopic methodology could separate the healthy people from the patients with exterior cold and interior heat, and the accuracy rate was 85.6%. This provides a new method for diagnosis of TCM syndromes. Based on normalized reflectivity treatment of the tongue spectrum of the healthy people and fatty liver patients, the accuracy rate of the classified pradiction of samples of the unknown healthy people and patients with fatty liver was 89.7%; using the same method to classify the samples of the unknown healthy people and hyperviscosity patients, the correct rate was 100%. The results show that tongue spectrum analysis can provide evidence for the diagnosis of disease.

利用光谱法测量的舌象信息非常丰富，但现有的方法研究也只是光谱所反映出来的信息，与中医整体观念、辨证论治等理论的结合还有众多问题需要解决。

The information of the tongue manifestation measured by the spectral method is very rich, but the existing method is only the information reflected by the spectrum, and there are many problems to be solved, such as its combination with the concept of holism and syndrome differentiation and treatment.

四、高光谱图分析法
4. Hyperspectral graph analysis method

高光谱图分析法，即光谱与图像结合进行分析的方法。采用推帚式的高光谱成像系统采集舌图，并使用基于 Gabor 滤波器的舌纹分析算法，对部分典型舌纹进行分类，结果表明高光谱舌象的分析方法明显优于传统的基于灰度图像舌纹的分析法。高光谱图分析法比光谱分析法更先进，更接近中医的传统理论，但在整合临床各种信息方面依然有待加强。

Hyperspectral graph analysis method is the method of combining spectral with image analysis. Using the high spectral imaging system of push broom to collect tongue graph, and using the tongue-pattern analysis algorithm based on gabor filter to classify some typical tongue pattern, the results showed that the analysis method of hyperspectral tongue manifestation is better than traditional analysis method based on gray-scale image tongue pattern. The hyperspectral graph analysis method is more advanced than the spectral analysis method, and is closer to the traditional theory of TCM, but it still needs to be strengthened in the integration of clinical information.

第三节　舌诊的客观化研究

Section 3　Objective Study of Tongue Diagnosis

一、计算机技术研究舌诊图像

1. Tongue diagnosis image based on computer technology

中医诊断存在一些模糊性问题，难以准确判定患者的状态，计算机、图像、光学技术的发展为解决这一问题提供了新思路。舌诊的图像信息处理始于 1986 年中国科学院合肥智能机械研究所和安徽中医学院的合作，研究者将《中医舌苔图谱》中的舌图转换为数字舌图，认为正常舌象与病理舌象之间红（R）、绿（G）、蓝（B）色度和灰度级数据存在明显差异。因此设想在标准光源条件下，将彩色摄像机拍摄的舌图转换为数字图像，通过对数字舌图的定量分析，建立以舌象色度变化分析为重点的数字舌图识别系统。另外，舌的物理特性主要反映在舌色上，舌象分析的前提应该是彩色图像的重现。为使得舌象在传送和显示过程中保持色彩的一致性和可重复性，进行色彩校正是很有必要的。近年来，随着数字摄像技术和色彩管理的发展，舌象色彩校正基本采用了数字技术。

There are some fuzzy problems in the diagnosis of TMC, so it is difficult to judge the condition of the patients accurately. The development of computer, image and optics technology provides a new way to solve these problems. The image processing of tongue diagnosis began in 1986 with the cooperation of Hefei Institute of Intelligent Machinery and Anhui College of Traditional Chinese Medicine. The researchers converted the tongue images in *The Tongue fur Atlas of Chinese Medicine* into digital tongue images, and found that the red (R), Green (G), Blue (B) color and gray level data were significantly different between normal tongue manifestation and pathological tongue manifestation. Therefore, it is envisaged to convert the tongue images taken by color camera into digital images under the standard light source, and to establish a digital tongue image recognition system focusing on the analysis of the color change of the tongue image through quantitative analysis of the digital tongue graph. In addition, the physical characteristics of the tongue are mainly reflected in the tongue color and the premise of tongue manifestation analysis should be the reproduction of color images. In order to maintain the color consistency and repeatability in the process of transmission and display, it is necessary to make color correction. In recent years, with the development of digital camera technology and color management, the color correction of tongue manifestation is mainly based on digital technology.

①基于计算机图像处理技术的舌色度量与诊断：舌象的直观性较强，众多学者对舌色进行研究。20 世纪 80 年代后期，孙立友等开始探讨利用计算机图像识别技术进行舌诊客观化研究，并对舌象的彩色图片进行探讨性试验。另外还有研究者使用"舌色仪"、计算机图像处理技术、舌诊综合信息分析系统等对正常人或患者的舌质颜色及 RGB 进行定量分析等。目前，舌色研究大体达到了一定的诊断符合率，也具有一定的参考意义，但它与临床病证只建立了简单的联系，并没有与其他舌象特征关联起来，因此临床应用受到了很大限制。

① Measurement and diagnosis of tongue color based on computer image processing technology: many scholars study the tongue color because the tongue manifestation is very vivid. In the late 80s of 20th century, Sun Liyou, etc. began to explore the objective study of tongue diagnosis by using computer image recognition technology, and conducted exploratory trials to the color picture of tongue manifestation. In addition, some researchers made quantitative analysis to the color of the tongue texture and RGB of normal people or patients by using "tongue colorimeter", computer image processing technology, and comprehensive information analysis system of tongue diagnosis. At present, tongue color research has reached a certain rate of diagnosis, and also has a certain reference significance, but it has only established a simple relationship with clinical syndromes, and has not been associated with other characteristics of the tongue manifestation, therefore, the clinical application has been greatly limited.

②图像分析技术与数据挖掘相结合的研究：将图像分析、网络、人工智能、数据挖掘等先进技术融合，建立开放式的舌象分析平台，使舌诊的客观化研究工作随着视觉技术、人工智能及模式识别等技术的发展而不断深入，促进图像处理与分析技术通过在中医领域的应用而得到新的认识；基于免疫聚类的 RBF 神经网络机等算法在舌

诊中的研究及应用，模型具有收敛速度快、识别能力强等特点；舌象分区训练识别法，即基于 AdaBoost 算法构建一套符合中医诊断体系的舌象分类识别算法，该方法已取得一定的分类识别效果；针对舌色和舌苔颜色的分类识别，提出基于 DAG 和决策树结合的方法，可在识别速度和识别率上有所提高。

② Research on the combination of image analysis technology and data mining: integrating image analysis, network, artificial intelligence, data mining and other advanced technology to establish an open tongue manifestation analysis platform, so that the objective study of tongue diagnosis deepens with the development of vision technology, artificial intelligence and pattern recognition technology, and promotes the new understanding of the image processing and analysis technology through the application in the field of Traditional Chinese Medicine. The research and application of RBF neural network algorithm based on immune clustering in tongue diagnosis, with the model's characteristics of fast convergence and strong recognition ability. The method of tongue manifestation partition training, which AdaBoost-algorithm-based is used to construct a tongue manifestation classification algorithm that accords with the traditional Chinese medicine diagnosis system, and has obtained some classification recognition effect. In terms of the classification and recognition of tongue color and tongue fur color, a method based on DAG and decision tree is proposed to improve the recognition speed and recognition rate.

二、舌诊仪研究

2. Study on tongue diagnosis instrument

中医舌诊是中医四诊客观化研究的重要内容之一。

Tongue diagnosis of Traditional Chinese Medicine is one of the important contents of the objective study of the four examinations.

①光源的选择：光源是获取客观舌象的重要外部条件，是舌诊成败的关键。建立光源采集保护装置，选择稳定性强、显色性好、接近传统舌象观察所需的自然光线的光源，可以使所获得的舌象信息更加客观、真实和稳定。目前，舌象信息客观化研究中所选择的光源的色温范围大多在 4500 ～ 6500K 之间。假如光源色处于人们所习惯的色温范围内，则显色性是光源质量更为重要的指标。这是因为显色性直接影响人

们所观察物体的颜色。Ra 值为 97 的德国 JUST 标准光源 D50 经科学实验证明是最佳选择。

① Selection of light source: light source is an important external condition to obtain the objective tongue image, and it is the key to the success of tongue diagnosis. Adopting light source acquisition and protection device, which has strong stability, good color rendering, and is close to the natural light source of traditional tongue observation, can make the acquired tongue information more objective, real and stable. At present, the color temperature range of the light source selected in the study of the information objectivity of the tongue manifestation is mostly between 4500-6500K. If the light source color is in the color temperature range which the people are accustomed to, then the color rendering is the more important index of the light source quality. This is because color rendering has a direct effect on the color of the objects that people observe. The German JUST standard light source D50 with the Ra value of 97 is proved to be the best choice by scientific experiment.

②舌象采集：舌象采集方法随着科学的发展和研究的深入不断改进，现在多采用舌象分析仪和采用暗室、国际照明协会（CIE）标准光源，规范照明角度、亮度及患者伸舌姿势等，分析仪当中使用数码或单反相机获得舌象照片，并通过简单的操作自动分析出舌象特征如舌色、苔色、苔厚、湿度、裂纹等信息来为我们的科研、教学服务。

② Tongue manifestation collection: the method of tongue manifestation collection has been improving with the development of science and the indepth of research. Nowadays, tongue manifestation analyzers, darkrooms, and the standard light source stipulated by International Lighting Association (CIE) are used to standardize the lighting angle, brightness, and the patient's tongue extension posture. The analyzer uses a digital or SLR camera to obtain tongue manifestation photos and, through simple operations, automatically analyzes the tongue manifestation's characteristic information, such as tongue color, fur color, fur thickness, moistness, fissure, etc., to meet the scientific research and teaching requirements.

③图像的校正与分割：舌象仪采集的舌图是在有固定光源的拍摄区域中获得，这往往与标准光源中所获得的舌图存在一定差别。为了让分析软件兼容各个光源下采集

的舌图，必须进行颜色校正，同时还包括舌体分割和舌质、舌苔的识别及区域划分等工作。这个过程是后续分析工作的基础部分。有研究基于颜色纹理的无监督图像分割法，利用色度参数调整后生成的模板进行区域匹配，并最终完成舌体的提取；有研究根据先验空间信息，利用多色彩通道动态选取阈值，提出分离舌质、舌苔的算法；利用舌图将超光谱图像立方体转换成光谱角度立方体，使二维的边缘检测转变成一维问题，简化了分割算法，且分割效果较好。

③ Image correction and segmentation: the tongue image collected by the tongue manifestation instrument is obtained in the shooting area with a fixed light source. There are some differences from the tongue image obtained with standard light source. In order to analyze kinds of tongue images under different light sources, color correction, tongue segmentation as well as recognition and regional division of tongue texture and tongue fur must be carried out. This process is the fundamental part of the follow-up analysis. Some unsupervised image segmentation based on color texture makes the region match with the template which is adjusted by chromatic parameter, and finally completes the extraction of the tongue. Some research based on the prior space information uses multi-color channel to select threshold dynamically, and proposes the separation algorithm of tongue texture and tongue fur. Using tongue graph to transform the cube of hyperspectral image into spectral angle cube, with two-dimensional edge detection transformed into one-dimensional problem, the segmentation algorithm is simplified, but the segmentation effect is better.

三、舌质的客观化研究
3. Study on objectification of tongue texture

在舌色方面，有研究者运用主要成分分析法，在 HSV 空间中提取舌象相关特征，通过 AdaBoost 算法解决舌色多分类问题，有效提高了分类精度；有研究者测定舌体 CDE 血流信号，运用腔内探头对异常舌象进行显像，通过血流像素网格化处理分析，对比正常和异常舌质之间的差异；有研究者采用舌质光谱分析原理，自制舌诊仪，用白炽灯光源的光束照射舌面，然后对反射光束分光处理和光电转换，用光强度反映色调、纯度与彩度信息。

In terms of tongue color, some researchers use the main component analysis method to extract the correlation characteristics of tongue manifestation in the HSV space, through the AdaBoost algorithm to solve the problem of multiple classification of tongue color and, thus, enhance the classification accuracy effectively. Some researchers measure the CDE blood flow signals of the tongue, use the cavity probes to show the abnormal tongue manifestation to compare the differences between normal and abnormal tongue texture through the analysis of the blood flow pixel grid treatment. Some researchers, with the analysis principle of tongue texture light spectrum and self-made tongue diagnosis instrument, use the light beam of the incandescent light to illuminate the tongue surface and then make light splitting treatment and photoelectric conversion to the reflected light beam, using the light intensity to reflect the information of hue, value and saturation.

在舌形方面，有研究者将舌色与纹理特征结合后，采用最优线性融合方法和 AdaBoost 算法，对舌象老嫩进行自动识别，结果基本满足识别要求。还有研究者将 RGB 分量转换为 HSV 分量，再用类间方差法确定阈值，并将各分量二值化，处理二值图像分割出舌体图，再进行图像开运算，最后运用凹点检测识别方法获得齿痕数。这种方法虽然能很好地获得齿痕数并区别程度，但对分割要求高，而且对轻度齿痕识别精度不够，有待进一步改进。

In the tongue form aspect, after combining the tongue color with the texture feature, some researchers use the optimal linear fusion method and the AdaBoost algorithm to automatically recognize the tongue manifestation's toughness and tenderness, with the result basically satisfied with the recognition requirement. Other researchers convert the RGB component to HSV component, use the inter-class variance method to determine the threshold value, binarize each component and process the binary image to segment the tongue body image for opening operation, and finally use the concave point detection and recognition method to obtain the number of tooth marks. Although this method can obtain the number of tooth marks and the degree of difference, the requirements for segmentation are high and the precision of the recognition of minor tooth marks is not enough. Therefore, it deserves further improvements.

在舌态方面，有研究者根据人体中轴线结合嘴角位置来判定舌体歪斜指数，实现对歪斜的定量分析；通过曲线拟合参数与曲线形状胖瘦的关系结合舌体长宽比，对舌体胖瘦进行定量分析。

In the tongue motility aspect, some scholars use the human body axis and the locations of the mouth corners to determine the deviation index of the tongue to achieve a quantitative analysis of deviated tongue. By analyzing the relationship between the curve fitting parameters and the curve shape, and the length-width ratio of the tongue, the quantitative analysis of the tongue body's plumpness and slenderness is conducted.

四、舌苔的客观化研究
4. Study on objectification of tongue fur

通过观察正常人舌黏膜超微结构的透射电镜和扫描电镜发现，健康人正常舌苔薄白苔是由丝状乳头分化的角化树与填充在其间的脱落上皮细胞、唾液、细菌、食物碎屑、渗出的白细胞等共同组成。舌苔的超微结构研究发现，3 个月的胎儿开始形成人类丝状乳头，其舌面无细菌附着；而成人舌苔则见表层角化剥落，并附有各种口腔细菌。各种病理舌象均可见大量细菌增殖。微生物学研究表明舌面是微生物寄居最密集、种类最复杂的部位之一，且每种细菌均占一定比例。

The transmission electron microscopy and scanning electron microscopy of normal tongue mucosa ultrastructure found that the normal thin white fur of healthy people is composed of the keratinized tree differentiated by filamentous nipples and the exfoliated epithelial cells, saliva, bacteria, food debris and exudation white cells etc. The ultrastructural study of tongue fur found that the 3-month-old fetus began to form human filamentous nipple with no bacterial attachment on the tongue surface while the adult tongue fur showed keratinized exfoliation of the surface layer and was accompanied by various oral bacteria. A large number of bacterial proliferation can be seen in a variety of pathological tongue manifestations. Microbiological research shows that the tongue surface is one of the place where there are the densest populations and the most complex species of microorganisms, and each kind of bacteria occupies a certain proportion.

结合中医理论探讨每种病理舌的微生物组成规律，有助于更清楚地阐明舌苔形成机制。

Using Chinese medicine theory to explore the microbial composition of each pathological tongue helps to better elucidate the mechanism of tongue fur formation.

在苔色方面，有研究者使用单色仪表示舌苔颜色的反射光波长，并排列成特定光谱，根据光源对应谱线获得舌苔的颜色组成。

In terms of fur color, some researchers use monochromator to show the reflected light wavelength of the tongue fur color, arrange them into a specific spectrum, and obtain the color composition of the tongue fur according to the corresponding spectral line of the light source.

在苔质方面，有研究者使用 Bayes 公式计算舌象的舌苔概率值来判断厚薄苔，结果显示，分布均匀的舌苔使用该方法效果较好，但当舌苔分布不均匀时偏差则较大；有研究者通过不同患者的舌苔涂片发现，凋亡相关基因（bax、TGF-β3）表达水平的变化可能是影响舌苔上皮细胞凋亡并导致舌苔厚度变化的重要原因；有研究者通过基于二分光反射模型中面反射、体反射理论的舌苔润燥分析法，根据润燥指数，将舌苔分为干、偏干、一般、略润、润、水滑等 6 级。此外，还有研究者通过使用"中医显微舌象仪"采取舌苔液样本，在显微镜下动态观察并统计不同证型标志物数量，探究舌苔液显微图的独特表现。

In terms of fur texture, some researchers use the Bayes formula to calculate the probability value of tongue fur to determine the thickness of the fur. The results show that this method is better for evenly distributed tongue fur, but the deviation is greater when the tongue fur is uneven. By observing the tongue fur smears of different patients, some researchers have found that changes in the expression levels of apoptosis-related genes (bax, TGF-β3) may be an important reason for the tongue fur epithelial cell apoptosis and the changes in tongue fur thickness. Some researchers have divided tongue fur into 6 grades according to the tongue fur moist-dryness analysis method and its index: dry, slightly dry, moderate, slightly moist, moist, water-slippery. And the tongue fur moist-dryness analysis method is based on the theory of surface reflection and body reflection in the binary light reflection model. In addition, some researchers took samples of tongue fur fluid by using the "TCM microscopic tongue manifestation instrument", dynamically observed and counted the marker number of different syndrome types under the microscope to explore the uniqueness of the tongue fur micrographs.

刘明等将高光谱成像技术用于中医舌诊舌苔信息的提取，发现高光谱技术在中医舌苔信息提取方面具有一定的可行性，能够为中医舌诊舌苔分离以及舌苔信息提取提供一种快速、简便的检测手段，为中医舌诊的客观化研究提供方法指导。

Liu Ming, et al. applied hyperspectral imaging technology to the extraction of tongue fur information in TCM tongue diagnosis, and found that hyperspectral technology has certain feasibility in the extraction, which can provide a fast and convenient detection method for the separation and information extraction of tongue fur, and offer methodological guidance for the objective research of TCM tongue diagnosis.

参考文献
References

［1］丁成华，孙晓刚.中医舌诊图谱·中英对照［M］.北京.人民卫生出版社，2003：1.

［1］Ding Chenghua, Sun Xiaogang. Tongue Figure in Traditional Chinese Medicine (Chinese-English)［M］. Beijing: People's Medical Publishing House, 2003: 1.

［2］许颖，曾常春，蔡修宇，等.原发性肝癌不同中医证型患者舌色的光谱测色及其色度学比较研究［J］.中西医结合学报，2012，10（11）：1263-1271.

［2］Xu Ying, Zeng Changchun, Cai Xiuyu, et al. Chromaticity and Optical Spectrum Colorimetry of the Tongue Color in Different Syndromes of Primary Hepatic Carcinoma［J］. Journal of Chinese Integrative Medicine, 2012, (11): 1263-1271.

［3］赵丰润.乙型肝炎肝硬化代偿期患者中医干预前后舌色参数变化特点的研究［D］.北京：北京中医药大学，2015：80.

［3］Zhao Fengrun. Study on the Change of Tongue Color Parameters Before and After Chinese Medicine Intervention in Patients With Compensatory Stage of Hepatitis B Cirrhosis［D］. Beijing University of Traditional Chinese Medicine, 2015: 80.

［4］宫爱民，曹玉，董秀娟，等.120例肝纤维化患者舌面象特征分析［J］.世界科学技术－中医药现代化，2016，18（10）：1646-1651.

［4］Gong Aimin, Cao Yu, Dong Xiujuan, et al. Analysis of Tongue and Facial Complexions in 120 Patients With Hepatic Fibrosis Based on the Parameter Characteristics［J］. World Science and Technology/Modernization of Traditional Chinese Medicine and Materia Medica, 2016, (10): 1646-1651.

［5］贾梓,郝建梅.舌下络脉积分与肝纤维化程度的相关性研究［J］.光明中医,2016,31（21）：3111-3112.

［5］Jia Zi, Hao Jianmei. Correlation Between Sublingual Vessel and Liver Fibrosis［J］. Guangming Journal of Chinese Medicine, 2016, (21): 3111-3112.

［6］宋铭悦.舌象的动态变化与慢重肝肝胆湿热证患者预后指标的相关性研究［D］.济南：山东中医药大学，2013：18.

［6］Song Mingyue. The Correlational Study Between the Dynamic Changes of Tongue Manifestation and the Prognostic Indicator of Patients With the Syndrome of Damp-heat in the Liver and Gallbladder of Chronic Severe Hepatitis［D］. Jinan: Shandong University of Traditional Chinese Medicines, 2013:18.

［7］李晓东，高秀娟，王蕾．舌诊在冠心病诊治中的应用体会［J］．河北中医，2014，36（7）：1015-1017.

［7］Li Xiaodong, Gao Xiujuan, Wang Lei. Application of Tongue Diagnosis in Diagnosis and Treatment of Coronary Heart Disease［J］. Hebei TCM, 2014, (7): 1015-1017.

［8］徐学功，张理，徐汴玲，等．慢性心衰患者证型及舌象分布特点与心功能分级的相关性研究［J］．北京中医药大学学报，2012，35（5）：312-316.

［8］Xu Xuegong, Zhang Li, Xu Bianling, et al. Correlation Between Distribution Features of Syndrome Types and Tongue Manifestations and Cardiac Functional Grading in Patients With Chronic Heart Failure［J］. Journal of Beijing University of Traditional Chinese Medicine, 2012, (5): 312-316.

［9］赵志宏．不稳定型心绞痛重度心气虚证舌象分析［J］．中西医结合心脑血管病杂志，2014，12（2）：241.

［9］Zhao Zhihong. Tongue Image Analysis of Severe Heart-qi Deficiency Syndrome of Unstable Angina Pectoris［J］. Journal of Integrated Chinese and Western Medicine with Cardio Cerebrovascular Disease, 2014, 12(2): 241.

［10］杨忠奇．基于"心开窍于舌"探讨冠心病（痰浊证）与舌苔菌群的相关性［D］．广州：广州中医药大学，2016：17-22.

［10］Yang Zhongqi. The Study of the Correlation Between Coronary Heartdisease (Phlegm Turbidity Syndrome) and Bacterials in Tongue Fur According to "Heart Opens into the Tongue"［D］. Guangzhou: Guangzhou University of Chinese Medicine, 2016: 17-22.

［11］史益平．舌质与冠心病相关性研究［J］．中医临床研究，2017，（9）：37-38.

［11］Shi Yiping. Research on the Relationship Between Tongue Quality and CHD［J］. Clinical Journal of Chinese Medicine, 2017, (9): 37-38.

［12］邓露露，丁成华，孙悦，等．淡白舌临床表征及意义探讨［J］．中华中医药杂志，2015，（8）：2699-2701.

［12］Deng Lulu, Ding Chenghua, Sun Yue, et al. The Application of Tongue Diagnosis in the Diagnosis and Treatment of Chronic Gastritis［J］. China Journal of Traditional Chinese Medicine and Pharmacy, 2015 (8): 2699-2701.

［13］吴耀南，苏晓芸．慢浅表性胃炎与舌象的相关性研究［J］．光明中医，2012，（3）：608-

611.

［13］Wu Yaonan, Su Xiaoyun. Study on the Correlation Between Chronic Superficial Gastritis and Tongue Picture［J］. Guangming Journal of Chinese Medicine, 2012, (3): 608-611.

［14］方华珍，丁成华，王玉臣，等 . 舌诊在慢性萎缩性胃炎辨证中的意义［J］. 中国中医基础医学杂志，2013，（4）：416-418.

［14］Fang Huazhen，Ding Chenghua, Wang Yucheng, et al. Tongue Diagnosis Significance in Syndrome Differentiation of Chronic Atrophic Gastritis.［J］. Tongue significance in syndrome differentiation of chronic atrophic gastritis, 2013, (4): 416-418.

［15］卢亚娟 . 腻苔在脾胃病中的临床意义［J］. 黑龙江医学，2014，38（9）：1084-1085.

［15］Lu Yajuan. Clinical Significance of Greasy Fur in Spleen and Stomach Disease［J］. Hei long jiang Medical Journal, 2014, 38(9): 1084-1085.

［16］安云霞，王雪峰，刘芳，等 . 小儿肺炎痰热闭肺证中舌象与肺部啰音变化的关系［J］. 中医儿科杂志，2012，（2）：23-25.

［16］An Yunxia，Wang Xuefeng，Liu Fang, et al. Relationship Between Tongue Manifestations and Pulmonary Rales in the Cases With Phlegm-Heat Blocking Lung Syndrome of Pediatric Pneumonia［J］. Journal of Pediatrics of Traditional Chinese Medicine, 2012, (2): 23-25.

［17］张淑琴 . 小儿肺炎风热闭肺证舌象变化的临床研究［D］. 大连：大连医科大学，2013：18-19.

［17］Zhang Shuqin. Clinical Study of Tongue Image in Wind-Heat Disturbing Lung Syndrome of Pediatric Pneumonia［D］. Dalian: Dalian Medical University, 2013: 18-19.

［18］戴芳，唐亚平，贾微，等 . 肺与舌象相关性的研究［J］. 中华中医药杂志，2012，（6）：1494-1496.

［18］Dai Fang, Tang Yaping, Jia Wei, et al. Study of the Correlation Between Lung and Tongue Manifestation［J］. China Journal of Traditional Chinese Medicine and Pharmacy, 2012, (6): 1494-1496.

［19］苏婉，许家佗，屠立平，等 . 207 例肺癌患者舌象在不同临床因素中分布规律研究［J］. 中华中医药学刊，2015，（11）：2703-2706.

［19］Su Wan, Xu Jiatuo, Tu Liping, et al. Study on Correlation Between Different Clinical Factors and Tongue Image in 207 Cases of Lung Cancer Patients［J］. Chinese Archives of Traditional Chinese Medicine, 2015, (11): 2703-2706.

［20］高振，李风森，荆晶，等 . 新疆和内地慢性阻塞性肺疾病舌脉特点的对比研究［J］. 中

华中医药杂志，2014，（8）：2626-2630.

［20］Gao Zhen, Li Fengsen, Jing Jing, et al. Comparison of Tongue and Pulse Characteristics of Chronic Obstructive Pulmonary Disease in Xinjiang and Inland Areas［J］. China Journal of Traditional Chinese Medicine and Pharmacy, 2014, (8): 2626-2630.

［21］张昱，翁维良，刘刚，等.慢性肾衰竭维持性血液透析患者瘀血舌与血清 hs-CRP 相关性的研究［J］.中国中医基础医学杂志，2010，16（10）：897-898.

［21］Zhang Yu, Weng Weiliang, Liu Gang, et al. Study on the Relationship Between Blood Stasis Tongue and Serum CRP in Chronic Renal Failure Patients with Maintenance Hemodialysis［J］. Chinese Journal of Basic Medicine in Traditional Chinese Medicine, 2010, 16 (10): 897-898.

［22］朱穆朗玛，张宇，金亚明，等.157 例慢性肾病患者不同肾功能分期的舌象特征研究［J］.世界科学技术－中医药现代化，2014，16（6）：1273-1277.

［22］Zhu Mulangma, Zhang Yu, Jin Yaming, et al. Research on Tongue Image Characteristics among 157 Chronic Kidney Disease Cases at Different Renal Function Stages［J］. World Science and Technology/Modernization of Traditional Chinese Medicine and Materia Medica, 2014 (6): 1 273-1 277.

［23］汤倩珏，陈锦黎，黎捷灵.肝郁肾虚型慢性盆腔炎舌象的观察研究［J］.中医当代医药，2010，17（15）：82-83.

［23］Tang Qianjue, Chen Jinli, Li Jieling. Tongue Manifestation characteristics of Chronic Pelvic Inflammation Patients With the Syndrome of Liver Depression and Kidney Insufficiency［J］. China Modern Medicine, 2010, 17 (15): 82-83.

［24］安鹏，何娜，吴喜利，等.肾病舌象客观化分析与辨证分型规律的探讨［J］.中国中医基础医学杂志，2013，19（2）：136-137.

［24］An Peng, He Na, Wu Xili, et al. Tongue Manifestation Objective Analysis and Syndrome Differentiation of Kidney Diseases［J］. Chinese Journal of Basic Medicine in Traditional Chinese Medicine, 2013, 19 (2): 136-137.

［25］诸凯，马一太.中医舌诊中的生物传热问题研究概况［J］.上海中医药杂志，2003，37（2）：58.

［25］Zhu Kai, Ma Yitai. Overview of Study on Biological Heat Conduction in TCM Tongue Diagnosis［J］. Shanghai Journal of Traditional Chinese Medicine, 2003, 37 (2): 58.

［26］李乃民，黄勃，刘珊，等.213 例厚形舌的临床观察［J］.中华中医药杂志，2008，23（2）：91.

［26］Li Naimin, Huang Bo, Liu Shan, et al. Clinical Observation on 213 Cases of Thick Tongues in Shape［J］. China Journal of Traditional Chinese Medicine and Pharmacy, 2008, 23 (2): 91.

［27］钱心如，陈泽霖，戴豪良，等.齿印舌的病理形态学研究［J］.中西结合杂志，1990，10（6）：337.

［27］Qian Xinru, Chen Zelin, Dai Haoliang, et al. Pathological Morphology Research on Tooth-Marked Tongue［J］. Chinese Journal of integrated Traditional and Western Medicine, 1990, 10 (6): 337.

［28］张旭，詹臻，蔡宝昌.表皮生长因子（EGF）对舌鳞癌细胞（Tca-8113）胞内钙离子的影响［J］.中医药学刊，2006，24（9）：1634.

［28］Zhang Xu, Zhang Zhen, Cai Baochang. Influence of the Epidermal Growth Factor (EGF) on Intracellular Calcium Ions of Tongue Squamous Cancer Cells (Tca-8113)［J］. China Chinese Archives of Traditional Chinese Medicine, 2006, 24 (9): 1634.

［29］邢锦绣，刘春霞，张惠平，等.舌诊与血液流变学的研究［J］.吉林中医药，1998，6（62）：56-57.

［29］Xing JinXiu, Liu Chunxia, Zhang Huiping,et al.The Research of Tongue Diagnosis and Blood Rheology［J］. Jilin Journal of Traditional Chinese Medicine, 1998, 6 (62): 56-57.

［30］魏学琴，张泉，韦虹，等.幽门螺旋杆菌与慢性胃炎的舌质、舌苔关系的分析［J］.成都中医药大学学报，1999，17（11）：7.

［30］Wei Xueqin, Zhang Quan, Wei Hong, et al. Correlation Betweenthe Tongue Texture and Tongue Coating of Chronic Gastritis and Helicobacter Pylori［J］. Journal of Chengdu University of Traditional Chinese Medicine, 1999, 17 (11): 7.

［31］沈英森，赵长鹰.白腻苔、黄腻苔与舌质的 pH 值及其临床意义［J］.湖南中医杂志，1995，11（5）：11.

［31］Shen Yingsen, Zhao Changying. PH Value of Tongue Texture with White Greasy Tongue Coating and Yellow Greasy Tongue Coating as Well as Their Clinical Significance［J］. Hu'nan Journal of Traditional Chinese Medicine, 1995, 11 (5): 11.

［32］王莉，秦吉华，迟永利，等.106 例胃癌患者舌苔脱落细胞观察［J］.山东中医学院学报，1995，19（4）：258.

［32］Wang Li, Qin Jihua, Chi YongLi, et al. Observation of 106 Cases of Exfoliated Cells of Tongue Coating in Gastric Cancer Patient［J］. Journal of Shandong College of Traditional

Chinese Medicine. 1995, 19 (4): 258.

［33］李新华, 吴正治, 周小青. 六种舌苔患者红细胞免疫功能及淋巴细胞 ANAE 活性观察［J］. 湖南中医药导报, 2000, 6（1）: 35-37.

［33］Li Xinhua, Wu Zhengzhi, Zhou Xiaoqing. RBC Immunologic Function and Lymphocyte ANAE Activity Observation in Six Kinds of Patients with Pathologic Tongue［J］. Hu'nan Guiding Journal of Traditional Chinese Medicine and Pharmacy, 2000, 6 (1): 35-37.

［34］吴正治, 李明, 张咏梅, 等. 常见舌苔上皮细胞 TGF-β3 基因表达特点的研究［J］. 中国中医药科技, 2003, 10（5）: 296.

［34］Wu Zhengzhi, Li Ming, Zhang Yongmei, et al. Research on Gene Expression Characteristics of Common Tongue Coating Epithelial Cells TGF-β3［J］. Chinese Journal of Traditional Medical Science and Technology, 2003, 10 (5): 296.

［35］吴正治, 李明, 张咏梅, 等. 常见舌苔舌上皮细胞凋亡及其相关基因表达研究［J］. 中国中医药科技, 2004, 19（2）: 98.

［35］Wu Zhengzhi, Li Ming, Zhang Yongmei, et al. Research on the Tongue Epithelial Cell Apoptosis of Common Tongue Coating and its Related Gene Expression［J］. Chinese Journal of Traditional Medical Science and Technology, 2004, 19 (2): 98.

［36］盛光, 吴正治, 李明, 等. 舌苔变化与凋亡相关基因分子机理的研究［J］. 中国中医药科技, 2005, 12（4）: 201.

［36］Sheng Guang, Wu Zhengzhi, Li Ming, et al. Research on Tongue Coating Changes and Apoptosis-related Gene Molecular Mechanism［J］. Chinese Journal of Traditional Medical Science and Technology, 2005, 12 (4): 201.

［37］李新华, 李晓荣, 吴正治, 等. 舌黏膜剥脱（剥苔）的基因分子机理研究［J］. 中国中医药科技, 2007, 14（4）: 233.

［37］Li Xinhua, Li Xiaorong, Wu Zhengzhi, et al. Research on Gene Molecular Mechanism of Tongue Mucosa Exfoliation (Peeledcoating)［J］. Chinese Journal of Traditional Medical Science and Technology, 2007, 14 (4): 233.

［38］贾海霞, 屈伸. 舌黏膜上皮 bax, bcl-2 基因表达与舌苔厚薄关系的研究［J］. 中国中医药科技, 2005, 12（3）: 176.

［38］Jia Haixia, Qu Shen. Relationship Between the Gene Expression of Tongue Mucosa Epithelial Bax, BCL-2 and the Tongue Coating Thickness［J］.Chinese Journal of Traditional Medical Science and Technology, 2005, 12 (3): 176.

［39］詹臻，吴慧平 . 表皮生长因子受体（EGF-R）放射受体分析方法（RRA）的建立［J］. 南京中医药大学学报，2001，17（4）：239.

［39］Zhan Zhen, Wu Huiping. Establishment of Radioreceptor Assay（RRA）of the Epidermal Growth Factor Receptor (EGF-R)［J］. Journal of Nanjing University of Traditional Chinese Medicine, 2001, 17 (4): 239.

［40］詹臻，汪红，王瑞平，等 . 舌苔与表皮生长因子（EGF）关系的临床研究［J］. 南京中医药大学学报，2003，19（1）：14.

［40］Zhan Zhen, Wang Hong, Wang Ruiping, et al. Clinical Research on the Relationship Between the Tongue Coating and Epidermal Growth Factor (EGF)［J］. Journal of Nanjing University of Traditional Chinese Medicine, 2003, 19 (1): 14.

［41］周坤福，詹臻，侯亮 . 表皮生长因子（EGF）影响舌苔形成的分子机制［J］. 南京中医药大学学报，2002，18（5）：283-285.

［41］Zhou Kunfu, Zhan Zhen, Hou Liang. Molecular Mechanism of the Effect of Epidermal Growth Factor (EGF) on the Formation of Tongue Coating［J］.Journal of Nanjing University of Traditional Chinese Medicine, 2002, 18 (5): 283-285.

［42］吴正治，李明，张盛薇，等 . 不同舌苔舌上皮细胞的凋亡及相关基因分子机理研究［J］. 中国中西医结合杂志，2005，25（11）：986-988.

［42］Wu Zhengzhi, Li Ming, Zhang Shengwei, et al. On Epithelial Cell Apoptosis of Different Tongue Coating and Related Gene Molecular Mechanism［J］. Chinese Journal of Integrated Traditional and Western Medicine, 2005, 25 (11): 986-988.

［43］方晨晔，唐志鹏 . 现代化舌诊在临床研究中的应用［J］. 中国中医药信息杂志，2016，23（6）：119.

［43］Fang Chenye, Tang Zhipeng. Application of the Tongue Diagnosis Modernization to Clinical Research［J］. Chinese Journal of Information on Traditional Chinese Medicine, 2016, 23 (6): 119.

［44］李谨，李媛 . 舌苔的光谱分析［J］. 陕西中医学院学报，2002，25（3）：67.

［44］Li Jin, Li Yuan. Spectral Analysis of Tongue Coating［J］.Journal of Shanxi College of Traditional Chinese Medicine, 2002, 25 (3): 67.

［45］应荐，沈雪勇，张志枫，等 . 乳腺增生病患者舌面各部红外辐射光谱比较［J］. 上海中医药大学学报，2006，20（1）：38-41.

［45］Ying Jian, Shen Xueyong, Zhang Zhifeng, et al. Comparison of Infrared Radiation

Spectra of Different Parts of Tongue Surface in Patients With Hyperplasia of Mammary Gland［J］.
Journal of Shanghai University of Traditional Chinese Medicine, 2006, 20 (1): 38-41.

［46］林凌，解鑫，李刚.基于光谱的中医舌色客观化方法初探［J］.光谱学与光谱分析，2009，29（3）：707-709.

［46］Lin Ling, Xie Xin, Li Gang. Spectrum-Based TCM Tongue Color Objectification Methods ［J］.Spectroscopy and Spectral Analysis, 2009, 29 (3): 707-709.

［47］林凌，张晶，赵静，等.基于光谱法的中医证型快速诊断［J］.光谱学与光谱分析，2011，31（3）：677-680.

［47］Lin Ling, Zhang Jing, Zhao Jing, et al. Spectrum-Based Rapid Diagnosis of TCM Syndromes［J］. Spectroscopy and Spectral Analysis, 2011, 31 (3): 677-680.

［48］严文娟，张晶，赵静，等.基于光谱法在中医舌诊疾病诊断中的应用研究［C］.中国中西医结合学会.第四次全国中西医结合诊断学术研讨会论文集.北京，2010：6-8.

［48］Yan Wenjuan, Zhang Jing, Zhao Jing, et al. Application of Spectral-BasedMethod to the Disease Diagnosis of TCM Tongue Diagnosis［C］. Chinese Association of the Integration of Traditional and Western Medicine. The Fourth National Symposium on the Diagnosis of Traditional Chinese and Western Medicine. Beijing, 2010: 6-8.

［49］李庆利，薛永祺，刘治，等.基于高光谱成像技术的中医舌纹分析算法［J］.光电工程，2007，34（4）：60-64.

［49］Li Qingli, Xue Yongqi, Liu Zhi, et al. Hyperspectral-Imaging-Based TCM Tongue Fissure Analysis Algorithm［J］. Opto-electronic Engineering, 2007, 34 (4): 60-64.

［50］孙立友，程钊，高逢生，等.利用计算机图像识别技术进行舌诊客观化研究的探讨［J］.安徽中医学院学报，1986，5（4）：5-7.

［50］Sun Liyou, Cheng Zhao, Gao Fengsheng, et al. Tongue Diagnosis Objectification Based on Computer Image Recognition Technology［J］. Journal of Anhui Traditional Chinese Medical College, 1986, 5 (4): 5-7.

［51］危小健，李明宏.“舌色仪”临床诊断初探［J］.南京中医药大学学报，1995，11（4）：13-14.

［51］Wei Xiaojian, Li Minghong. Preliminary Study of Clinical Diagnosis of Tongue Color Apparatus［J］. Journal of Nanjing University of Traditional Chinese Medicine, 1995, 11 (4): 13-14.

［52］刘庆，岳小强，邓伟哲，等.应用舌诊综合信息分析系统对原发性肝癌舌质颜色的定量

分析 [J]. 中西医结合学报, 2003, 1 (3): 180-183.

[52] Liu Qing, Yue Xiaoqiang, Deng Weizhe, et al. Quantitative Study on Tongue Color in Primary Liver Cancer Patients: Application of Comprehensive Information Analysis System of Tongue Diagnosis [J]. Journal of Chinese Integrative Medicine, 2003, 1 (3): 180-l83.

[53] 晏峻峰, 季梁, 施诚. 基于图像分析技术的开放式舌象研究平台的构建 [J]. 医学信息, 2004, 17 (1): 2-3.

[53] Yan Junfeng, Ji Liang, Shi Cheng. Construction of Open Tongue Manifestation Research Platform: Based on Image Analysis Technology [J]. Medical Information, 2004, 17 (1): 2-3.

[54] 谢铮桂, 韦玉科, 钟少丹. 基于免疫聚类的 RBF 神经网络在中医舌诊诊断中的应用 [J]. 计算机应用与软件, 2009, 26 (4): 42-43.

[54] Xie Zhenggui, Wei Yuke, Zhong Shaodan. Application of Immune-Clustering-Based RBF Neural Networks to TCM Tongue Diagnosis [J]. Computer Applications and Software, 2009, 26 (4): 42-43.

[55] 张萌, 胡显伟, 王元斌, 等. AdaBoost 算法在中医舌诊图像分区识别中的研究 [J]. 小型微型计算机系统, 2008, 29 (6): 1149-1153.

[55] Zhang Meng, Hu Xianwei, Wang Yuanbin, et al. Research on AdaBoost Algorithm in Tongue Manifestation Partition and Recognition of TCM Tongue Diagnosis [J]. Journal of Chinese Computer Systems, 2008, 29 (6): 1149-1153.

[56] 李晓宇, 张新峰, 沈兰荪. 基于支撑向量机的中医舌色苔色识别算法研究 [J]. 北京生物医学工程, 2006, 25 (1): 43-46.

[56] Li Xiaoyu, Zhang Xinfeng, Shen Lansun. Algorithm of TCM Tongue Color and Coating Color Recognitions: Based on Support Vector Machine [J]. Beijing Biomedical Engineering, 2006, 25 (1): 43-46.

[57] 陈雪姣, 王玉臣, 王德才. 中医舌诊客观化研究的发展概况 [J]. 江西中医药, 2012, 1 (43): 72-75.

[57] Chen Xuejiao, Wang Yuchen, Wang Decai. Overview of the Development of TCM Tongue Diagnosis Objectification [J]. Jiangxi journal of Traditional Chinese Medicine, 2012, 1 (43): 72-75.

[58] 王郁中, 杨杰, 周越, 等. 图像分割技术在中医舌诊客观化研究中的应用 [J]. 生物医学工程学杂志, 2005, 22 (6): 1128-1133.

［58］Wang Yuzhong, Yang Jie, Zhou Yue, et al. Application of Image Segmentation to TCM Tongue Diagnosis Objectification［J］. Journal of Biomedical Engineering, 2005, 22 (6): 1128-1133.

［59］陈海燕，卜佳俊，龚一萍，等．一种基于多色彩通道动态阈值的舌苔舌质分离算法［J］.北京生物医学工程，2006，25（5）：466-469.

［59］Chen Haiyan, Bu Jiajun, Gong Yiping, et al. Algorithm of Tongue Body and Tongue Coating Separation: Based on the Dynamic Threshold of Multiple Color Channels［J］. Beijing Biomedical Engineering, 2006, 25 (5): 466-469.

［60］胡申宁，李文书，施国生，等．基于 PcA-AdaBooat 的舌象颜色分类研究［J］.广西师范大学学报，2009，27（3）：158-161.

［60］Hu Kunning, Li Wenshu, Shi Guosheng, et al. Study on the Classification of Tongue Color: Based on PcA-AdaBooat［J］. Journal of Guangxi Normal University, 2009, 27 (3): 158-161.

［61］杨如芬，陈剑，李潇，等．舌彩色血流信号平均密度与中医舌质的相关性分析［J］.中国超声诊断杂志，2006，7（6）：406-407.

［61］Yang Rufen, Chen Jian, Li Xiao, et al. Correlation Analysis Between Mean Blood Flow Signal Density of the Tongue and TCM Tongue Texture［J］. Chinese Journal of Ultrasound Diagnosis, 2006, 7 (6): 406-407.

［62］严智强，王一中，李洪山，等．舌诊的物理分析—舌诊仪的研制及其临床观察［J］.贵州医药，1984，8（4）：1-3.

［62］Yan Zhiqiang, Wang Yizhong, Li Gongshan, et al. Physical Analysis of Tongue Diagnosis: the Development of Tongue Diagnosis Instrument and its Clinical Observation［J］. Guizhou Medical Journal, 1984, 8 (4): 1-3.

［63］曹美玲，张新峰，沈兰荪．分类器融合技术在中医舌象老嫩识别中的应用研究［J］.北京生物医学工程，2006，25（6）：644-648.

［63］Cao Meiling, Zhang Xinfeng, Shen Lansun. Application of Classifier Fusion Technique to the Recognition of Toughand Tender Tongue Manifestations［J］. Beijing Biomedical Engineering, 2006, 25 (6): 644-648.

［64］钟少丹，谢铮桂，蔡群英．齿痕舌识别方法的研究［J］.韩山师范学院学报，2008，29（6）：34-37.

［64］Zhong Shaodan, Xie Zhenggui, Cai Qunying. On the Identification Method of Teeth-Marked Tongue［J］. Journal of Hanshan Normal University, 2008, 29 (6): 34-37.

［65］龚一萍，倪美文．图像处理技术对舌诊客观化研究的进展［J］．浙江中医药大学学报，2007，3l（2）：242-244.

［65］Gong Yiping, Ni Meiwen. Review on the Application of Image Dealing Technology to Objective Study of Tongue Diagnosis［J］. Journal Zhejiang Chinese Medical University, 2007, 3l (2): 242-244.

［66］郭振华，王宽全．基于 Bayes 公式的舌苔厚薄分析［J］．中国医学物理学杂志，2004，21（6）：332-333.

［66］Guo Zhenhua,Wang Kuanquan. Identification of Tongue Coating Thickness: Based on Bayes Formula［J］. Chinese Journal of Medical Physics, 2004, 21 (6): 332-333.

［67］李明，潘文群，吴正治，等．厚苔形成与 bax、TGF-β3 基因表达及舌上皮细胞凋亡关系研究［J］．中医研究，2005，18（8）：19-21.

［67］Li Ming, Pan Wenqun, Wu Zhengzhi, et al. Relationship Between the Formation of Thick Tongue Coating and Bax, TGF-β 3 Gene Expression as Well as the Apoptosis of Tongue Epithelial Cells［J］. Traditional Chinese Medicinal Research, 2005, 18 (8): 19-21.

［68］蔡轶珩，沈兰荪．二分光反射模型在中医舌苔润燥分析中的应用［J］．电子学报，2004，32（6）：1026-1028.

［68］Cai Yiheng, Shen Lansun. Application of Dichromatic Reflection Model to TCM Moist-Dryness Analysis of Tongue Coating［J］. Acta Electronica, 2004, 32 (6): 1026-1028.

［69］王小满，杨必安，陈勇．中医显微舌像仪—苔液显微图像辨证初探［J］．中医杂志，2010，51：21-22.

［69］Wang Xiaoman, Yang Bian, Chen Yong. TCM Microtongue Imager: Syndrome Identification by Tongue Coating Excretion Micrograph［J］. Journal of Traditional and Chinese Medicine, 2010, 51: 21-22.

［70］刘明，赵静，李刚，等．高光谱成像用于中医舌诊舌苔信息提取［J］．光谱学与光谱分析，2017，37（1）：162-165.

［70］Liu Ming, Zhao Jing, Li Gang,et al. Application of Hyperspectral Imaging to Information Extraction of Tongue Coatingin TCM Tongue Diagnosis［J］. Spectroscopy and Spectral Analysis, 2017, 37 (1): 162-165.

［71］Ding Chenghua, Sun Xiaogang. Atlas of Tongue Dingnosis［M］. Beijing:People's Medical Publishing House, 2008: 4.